UP, DOWN, and ALL AROUND
the TYPE 1 DIABETES guidebook for kids

Written and illustrated

by

Amelia Pinegar

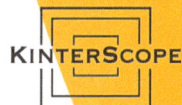
KINTERSCOPE

For Hyrum,
who knows what mimic means.

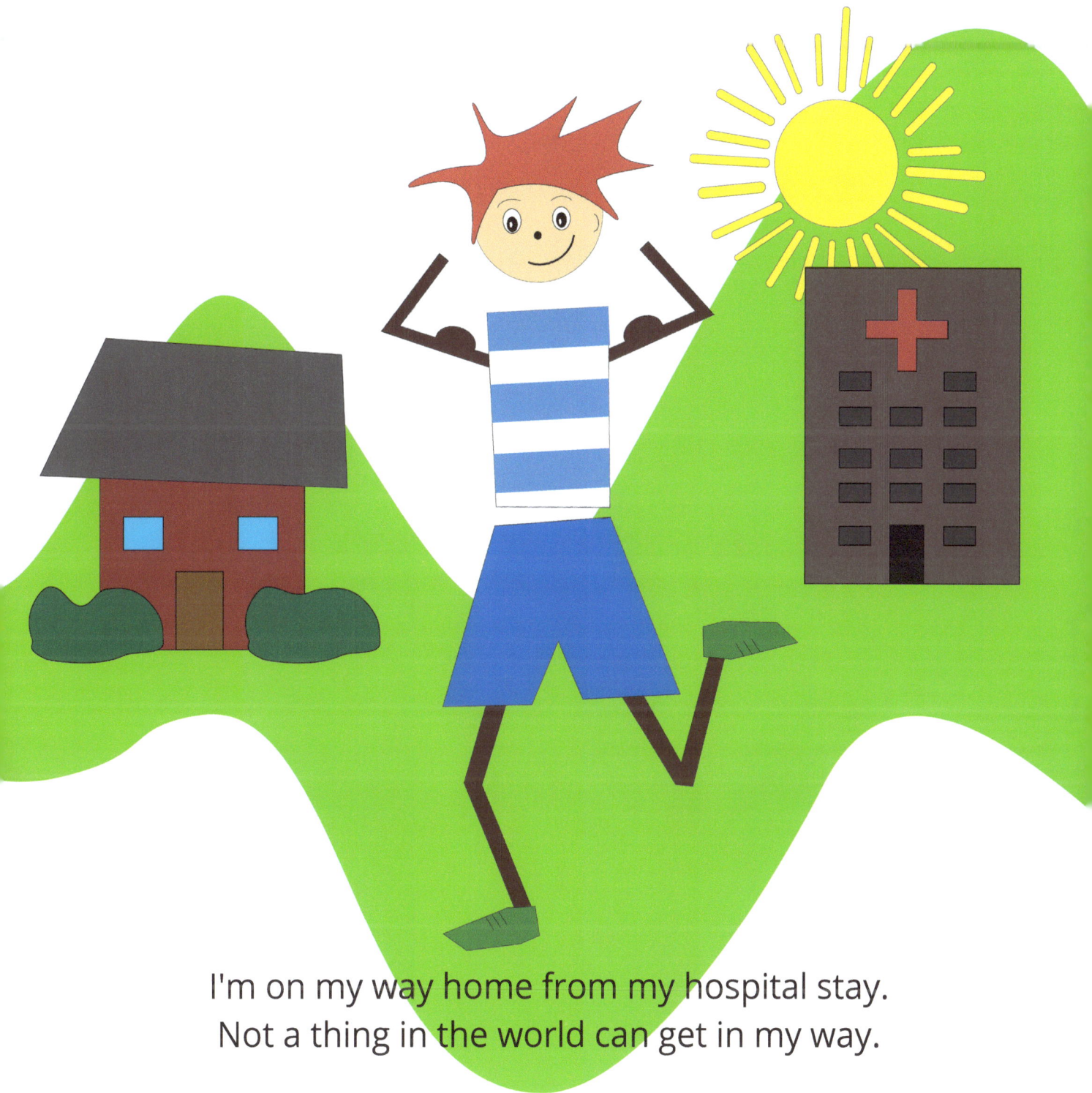

I'm on my way home from my hospital stay.
Not a thing in the world can get in my way.

I've got diabetes. But it won't get me.
Cuz I've got more smarts than a chimpanzee.

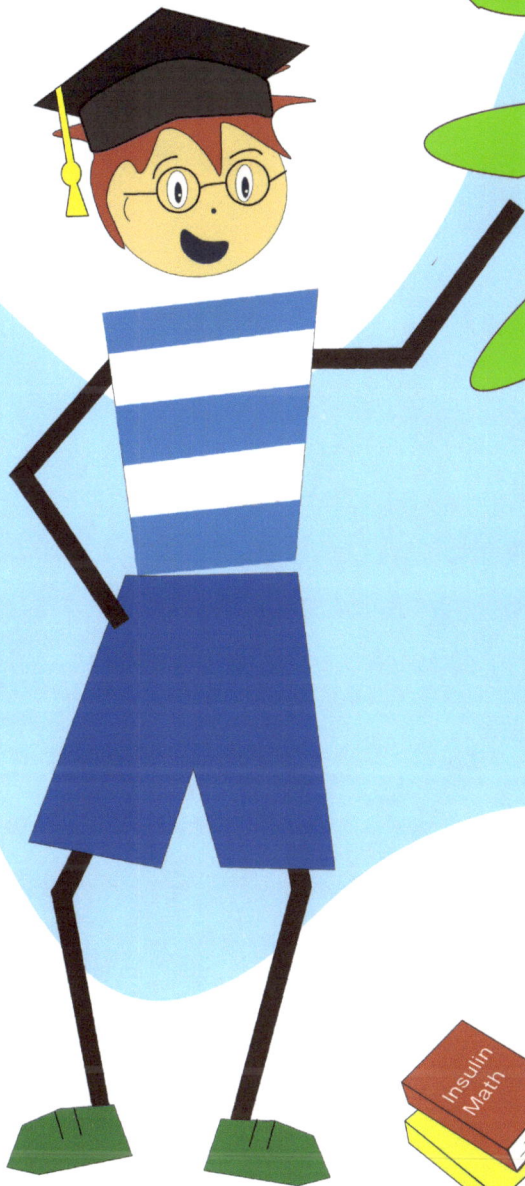

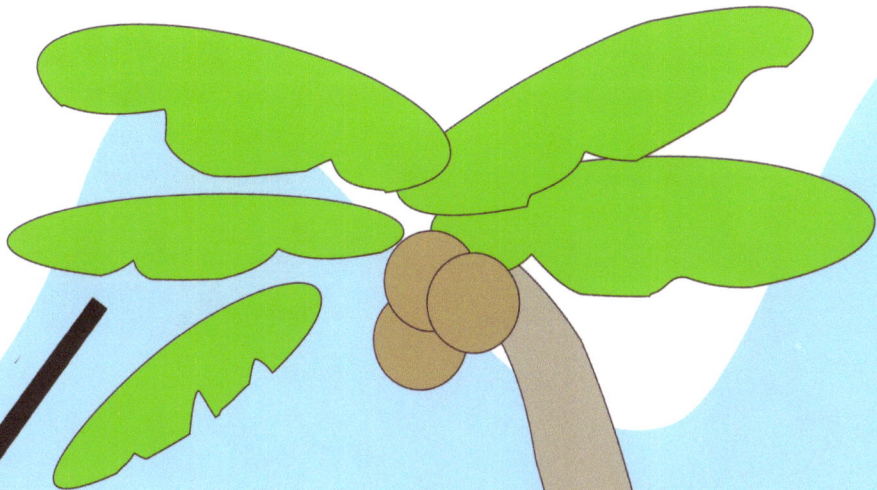

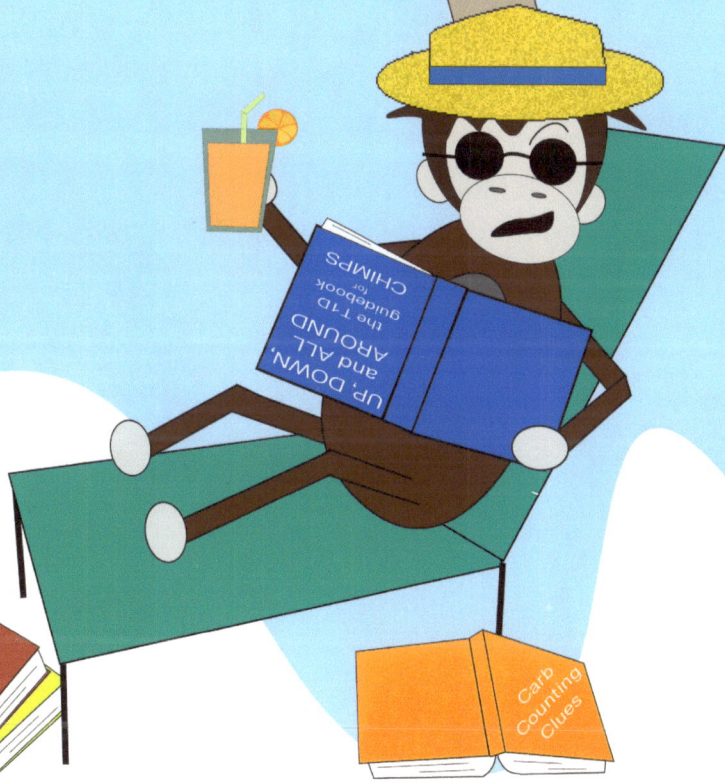

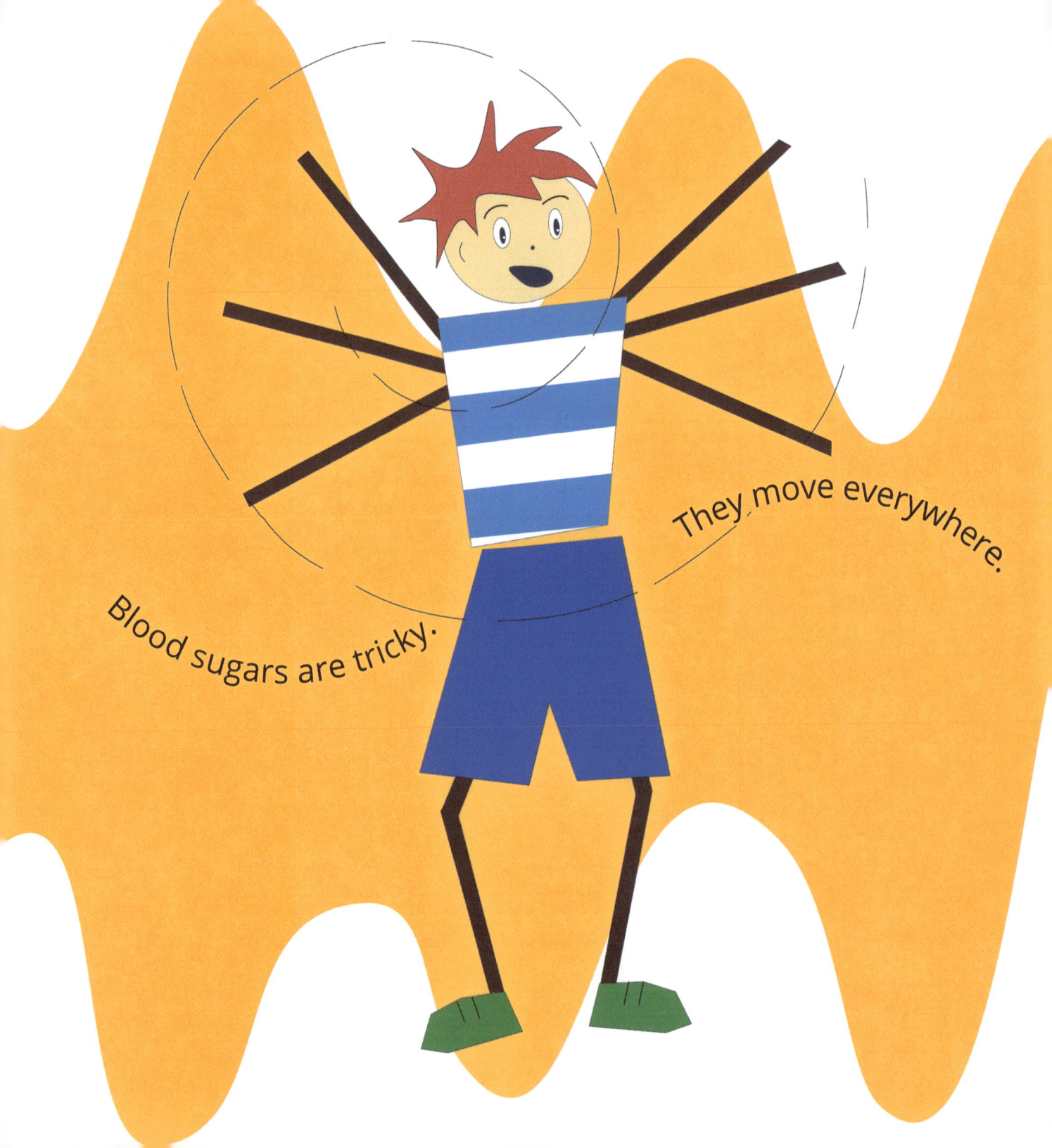

Blood sugars are tricky.

They move everywhere.

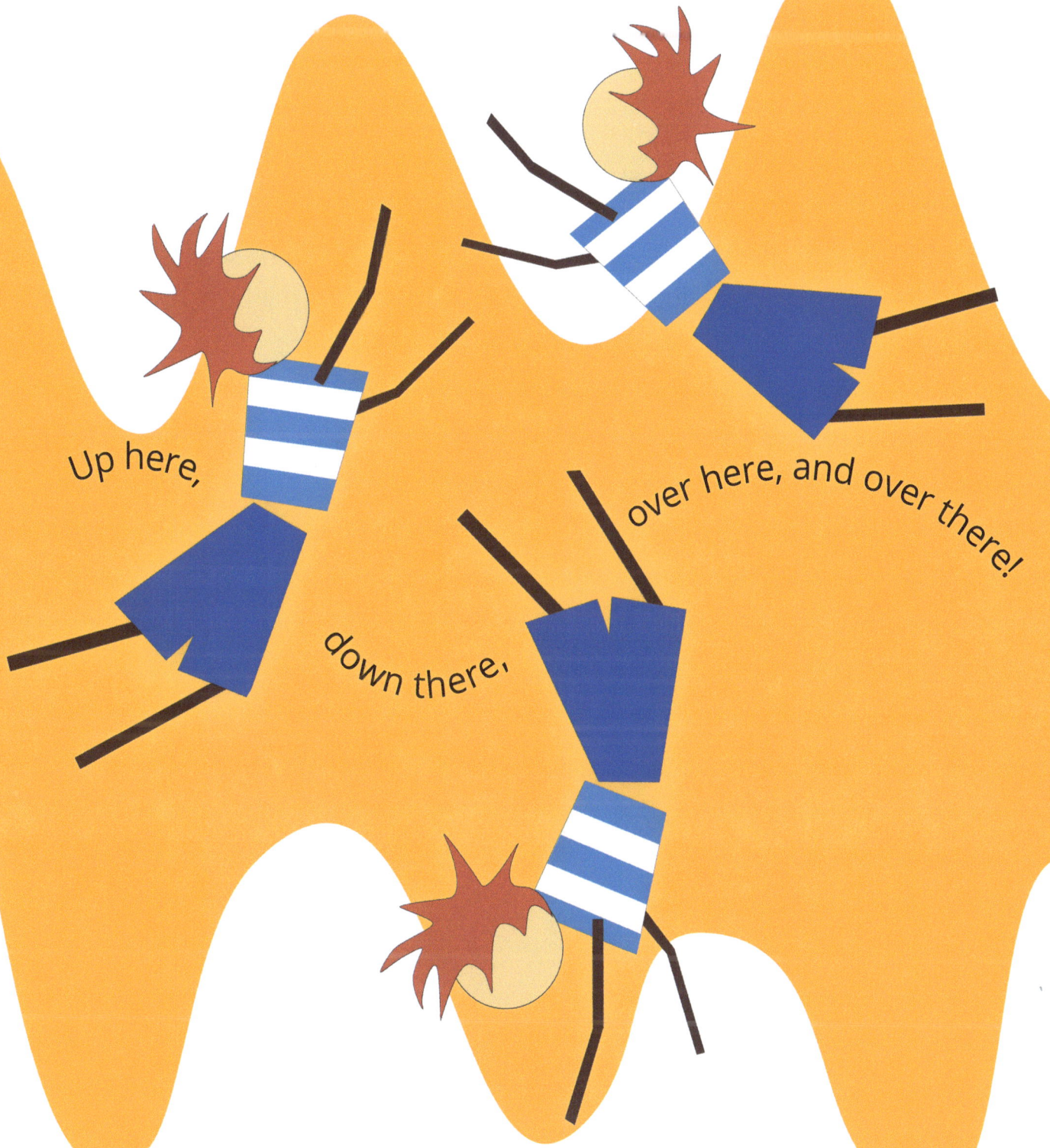

Up here,

down there,

over here, and over there!

Sooo...,
I've got all these tools right here in this pack.
It's my do-it-myself pancreas hack.

It holds all the things I need to survive.
Stuff that will help me and keep me alive.

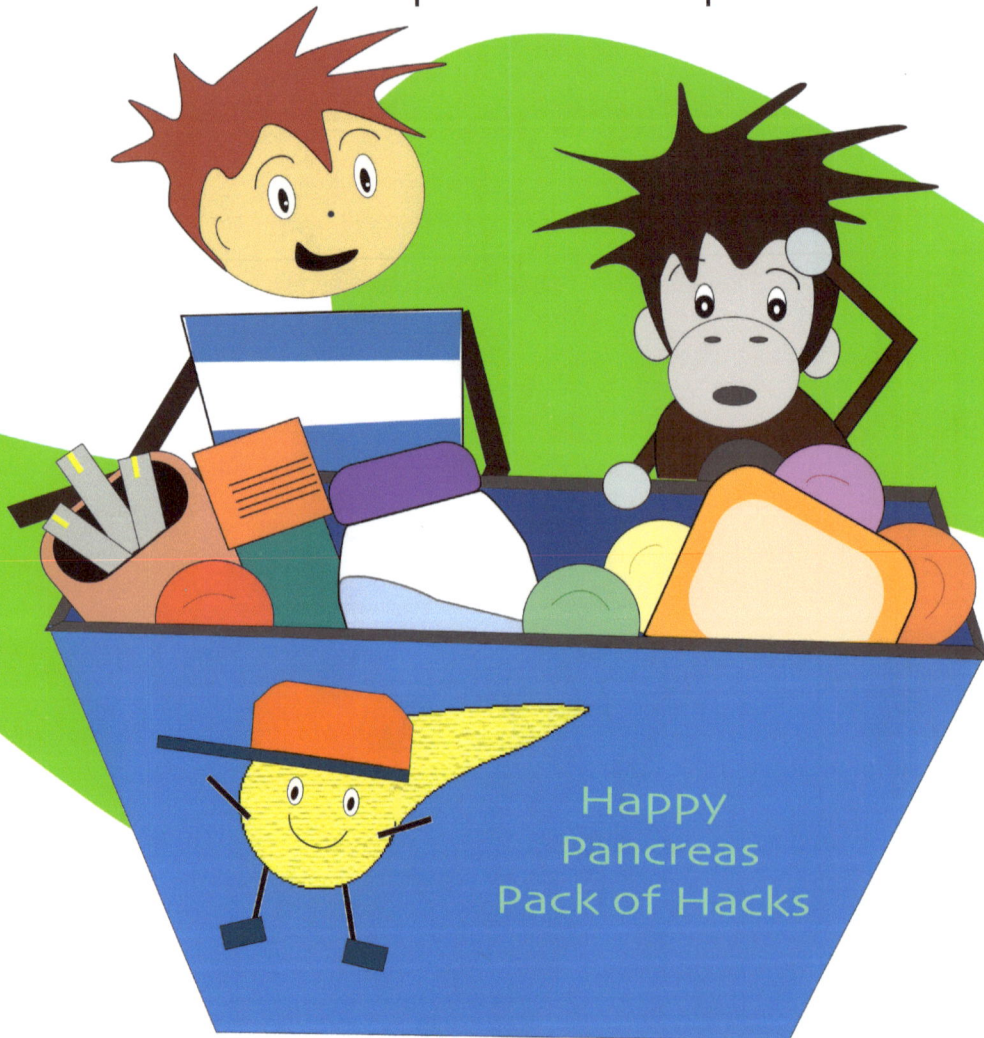

Happy
Pancreas
Pack of Hacks

First, there's this blood testing thinger-ma-ringer.
It reads my blood sugar right off my finger!

And tells me the info I need to know
to treat my sugars when I'm on the go.

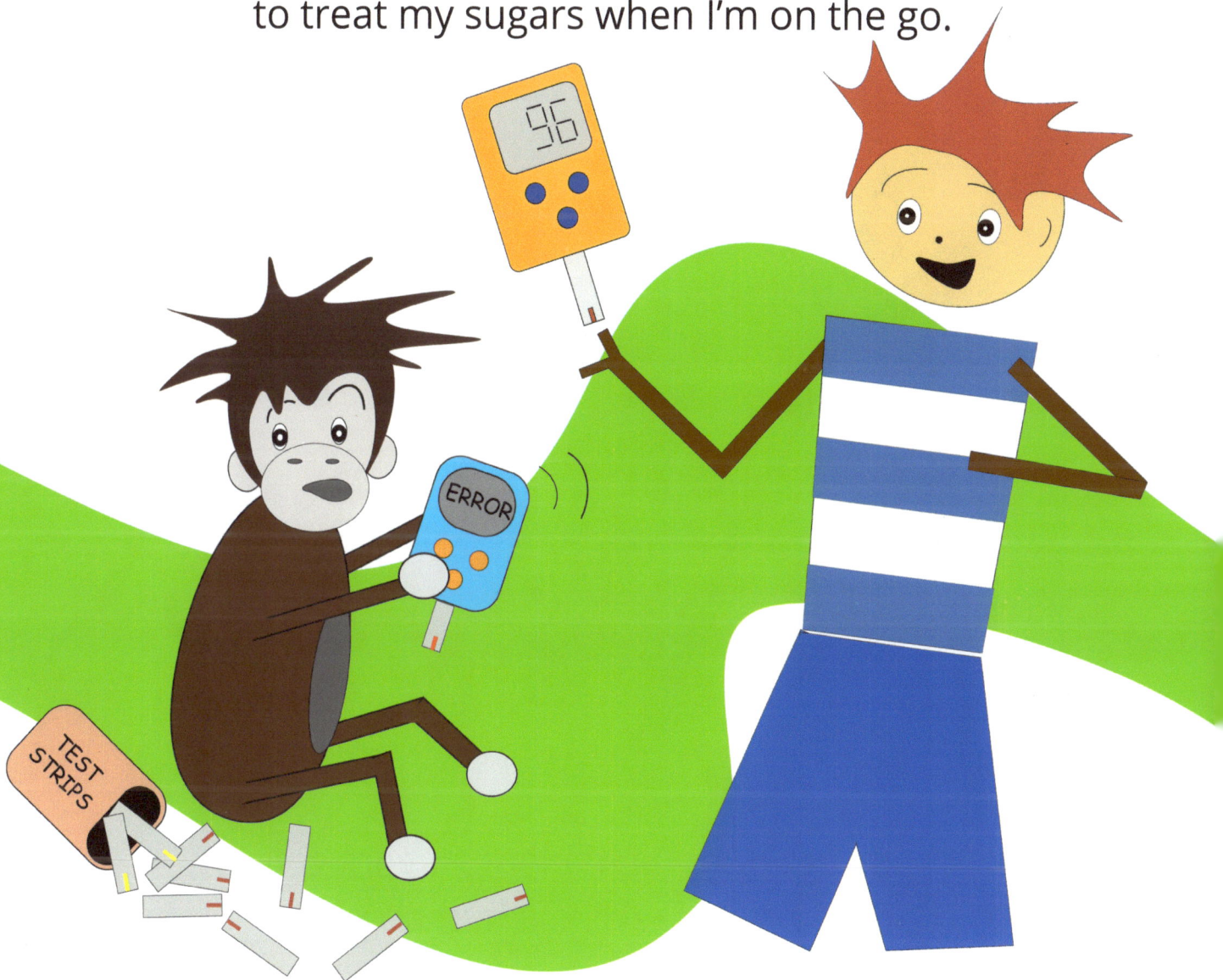

96

ERROR

TEST STRIPS

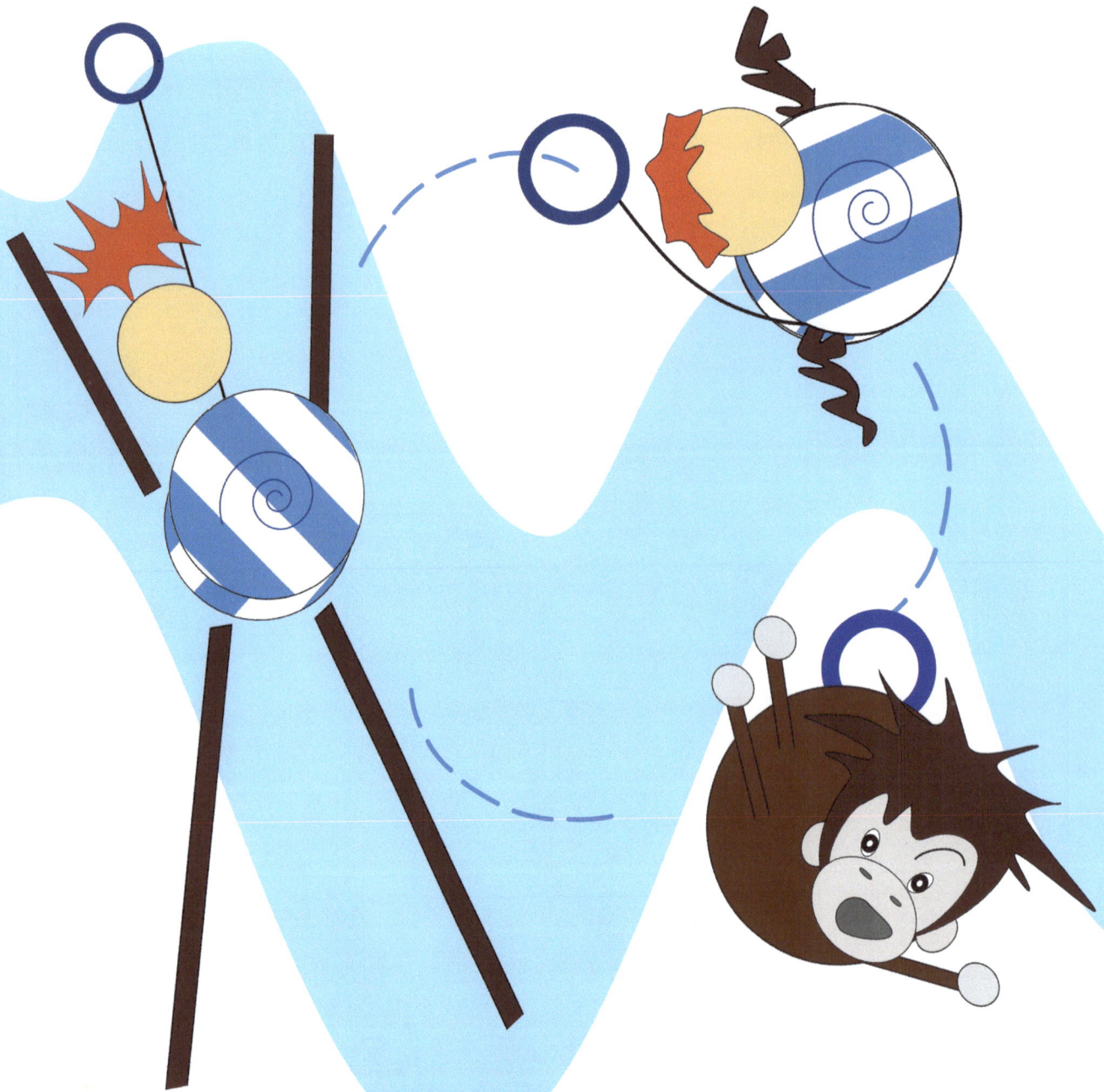

Blood sugars go high. Blood sugars go low.
Some days I feel like a human yo-yo.

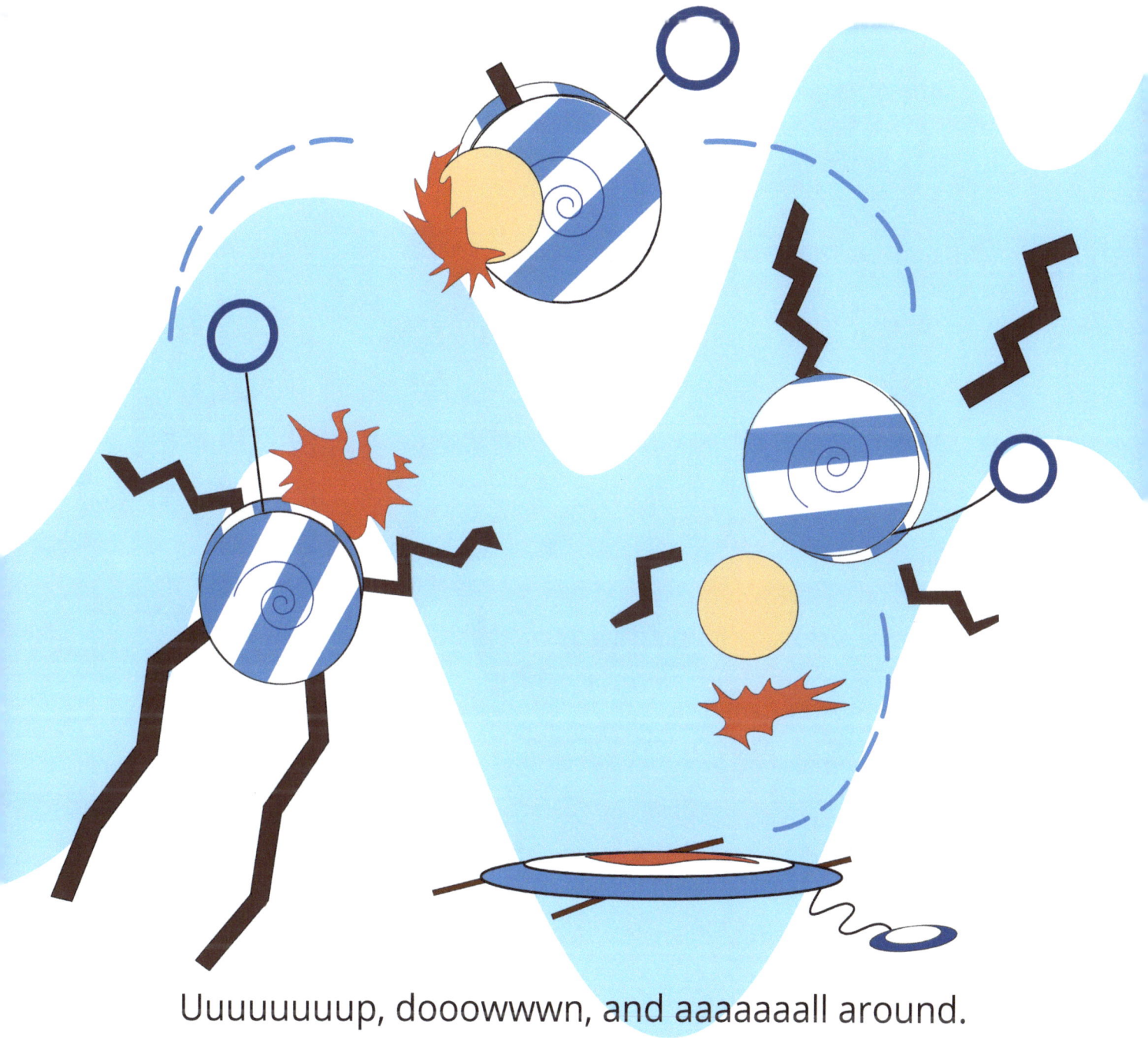

Uuuuuuuup, dooowwwn, and aaaaaaall around.
Sometimes I feel like I've crashed to the ground.

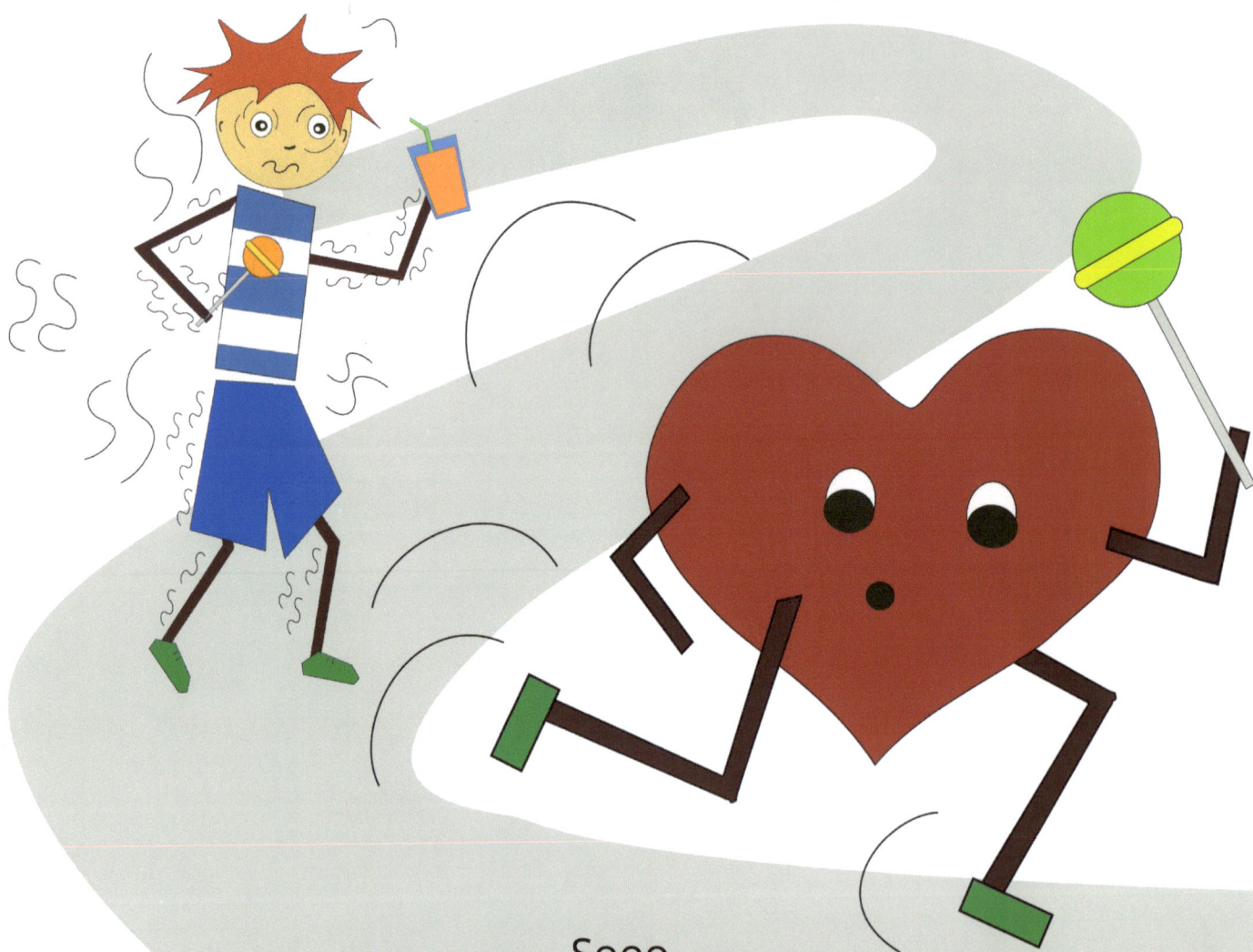

Sooo...,
I've got these carb snacks for when I'm hypo.
(That's fancy talk for blood sugar gone low.)

Hypoglycemia ain't no kind of fun.
It feels like the shakes with a heart on the run.

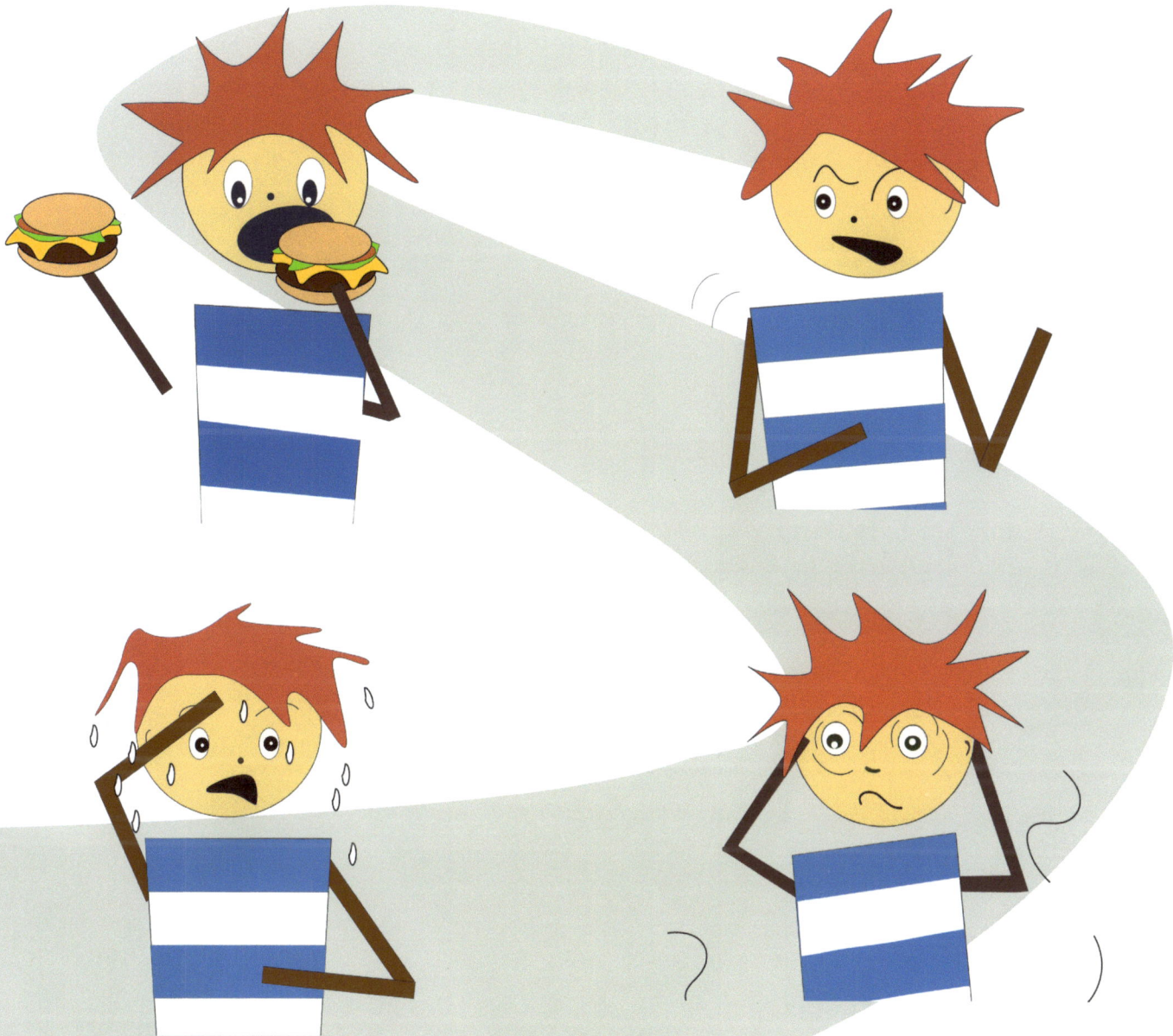

It also feels hungry, grouchy, and sweaty.
If it lasts too long, I start to get fretty.

So, the carbs are very important, you see,
to bring me back up to the me that is me.

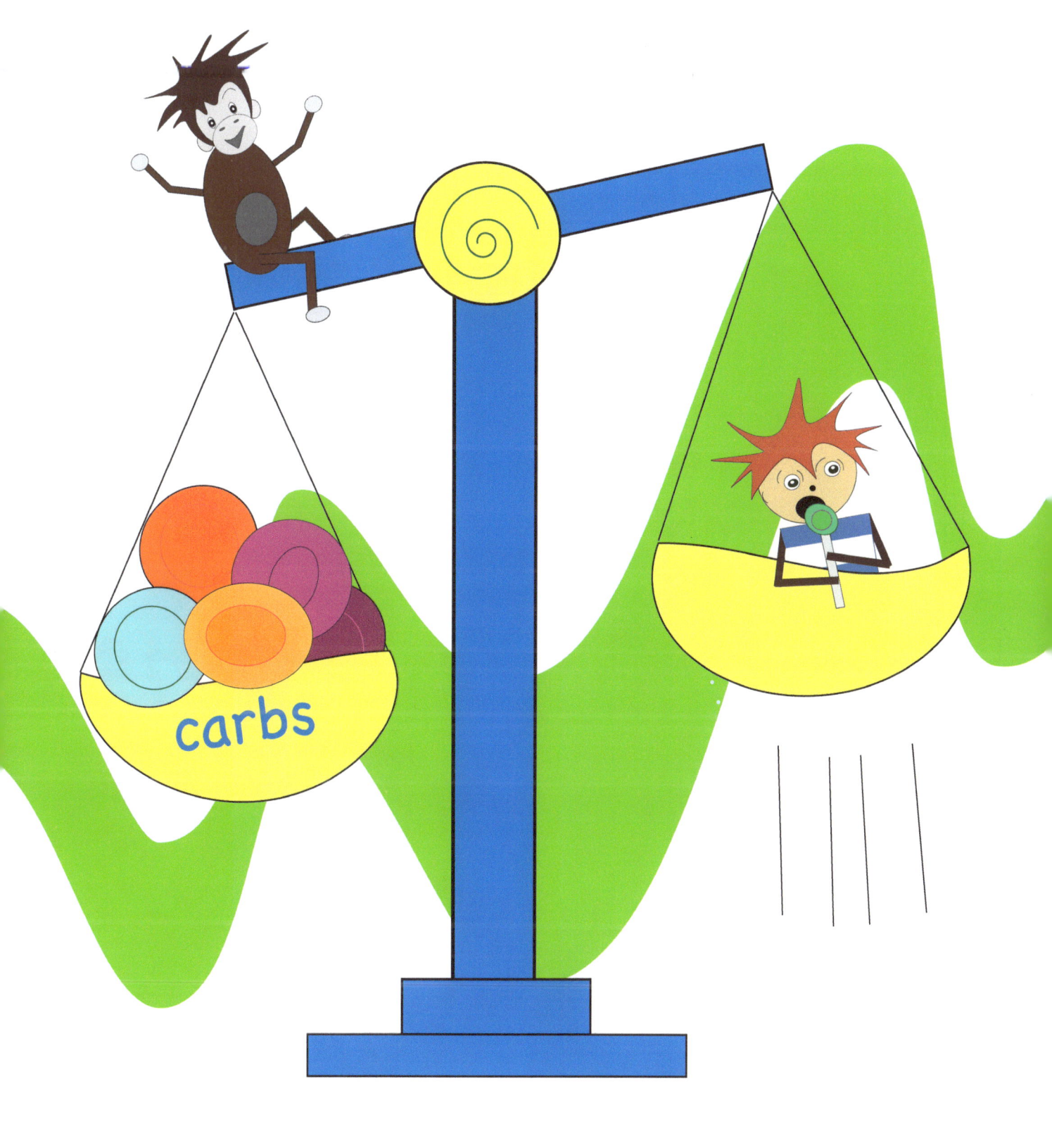

carbs

What is a carb snack? I'm so glad you asked!
Carbs are sugars you can eat in a flash!

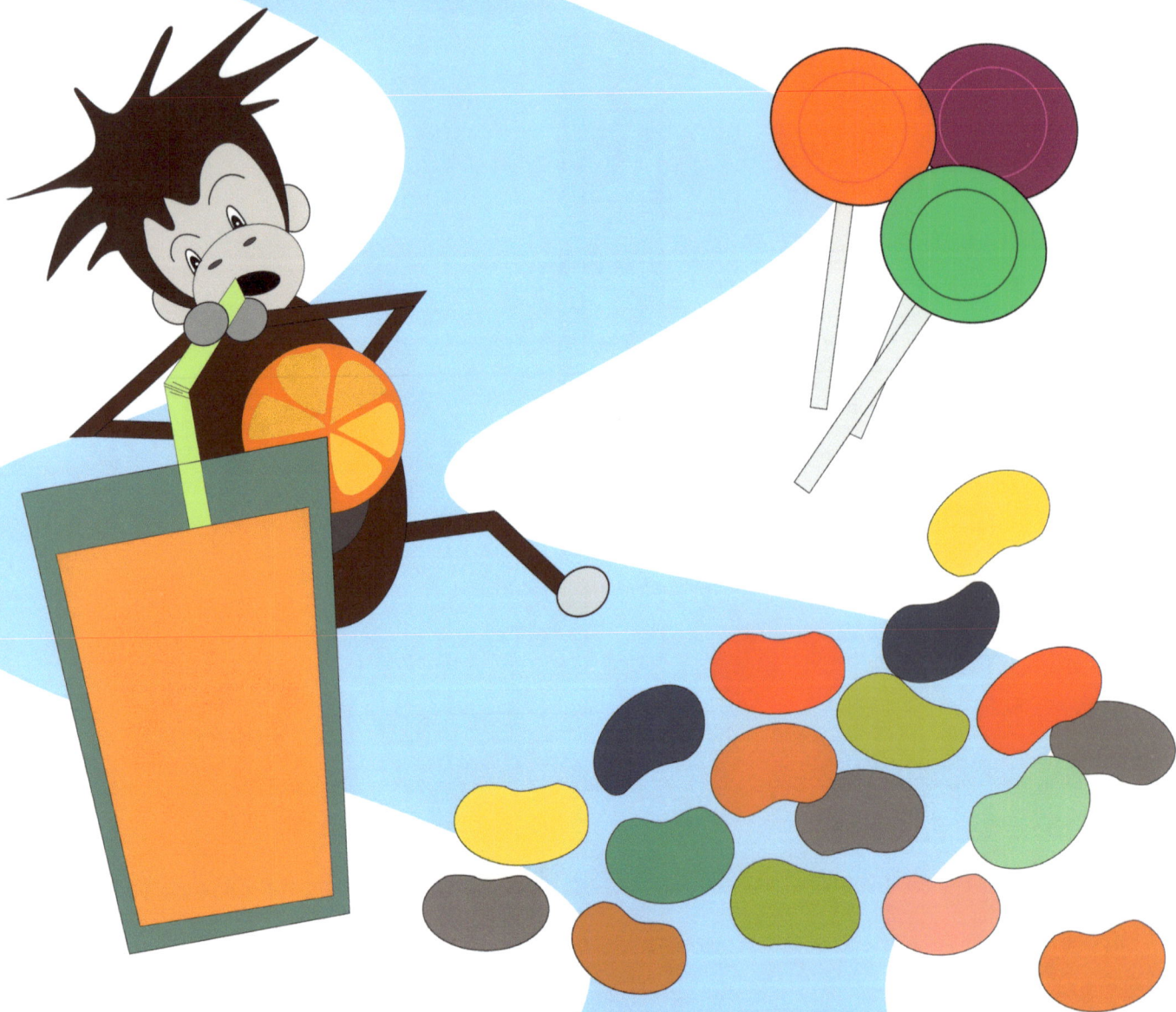

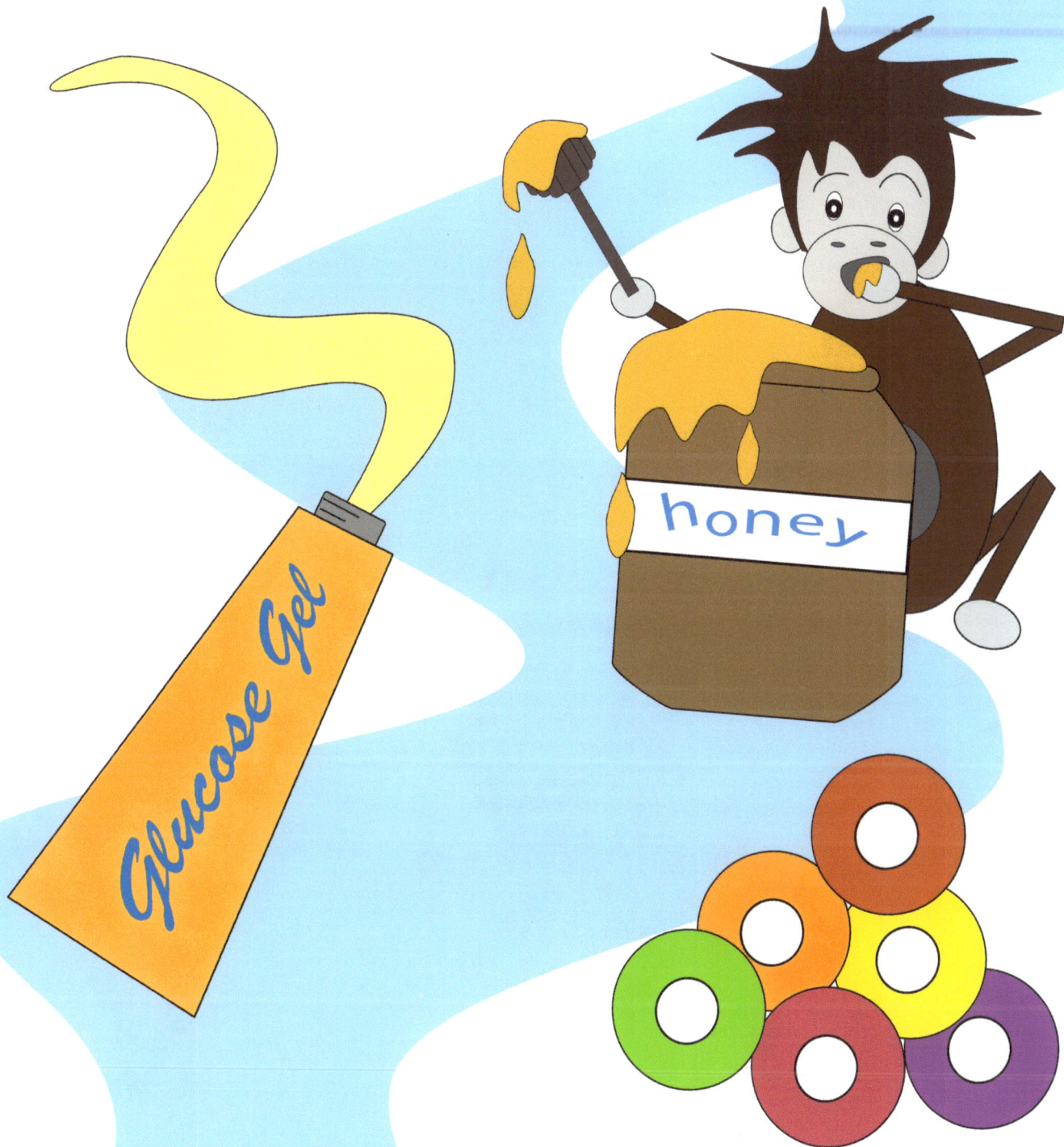

Blood sugars go low. Blood sugars go high. Some days it feels like a carnival ride.

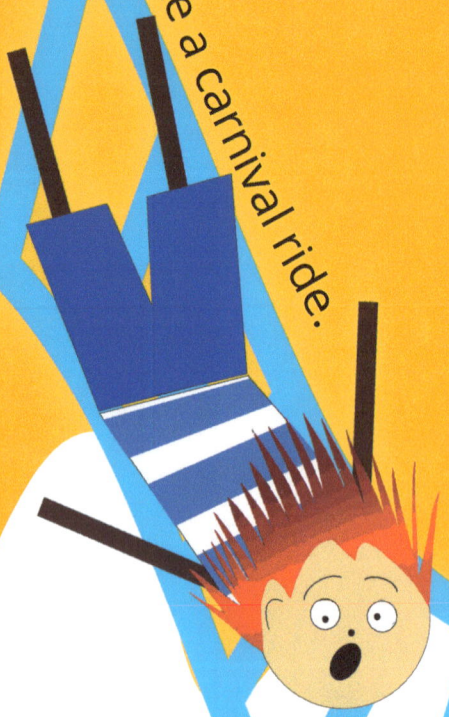

Uuuuuuuuuup, doooowwwn, and aaaaaall around.

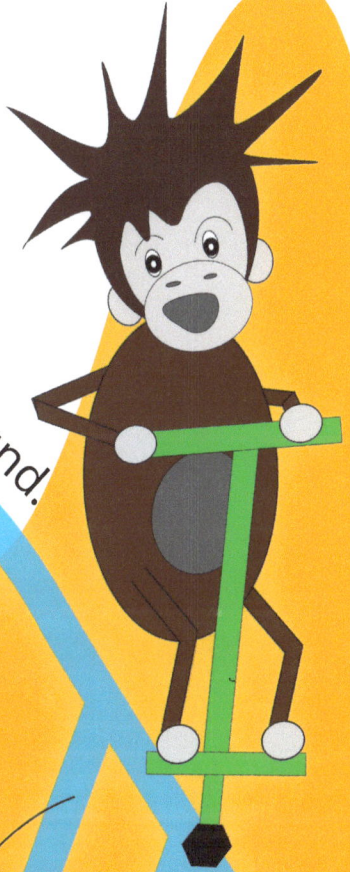

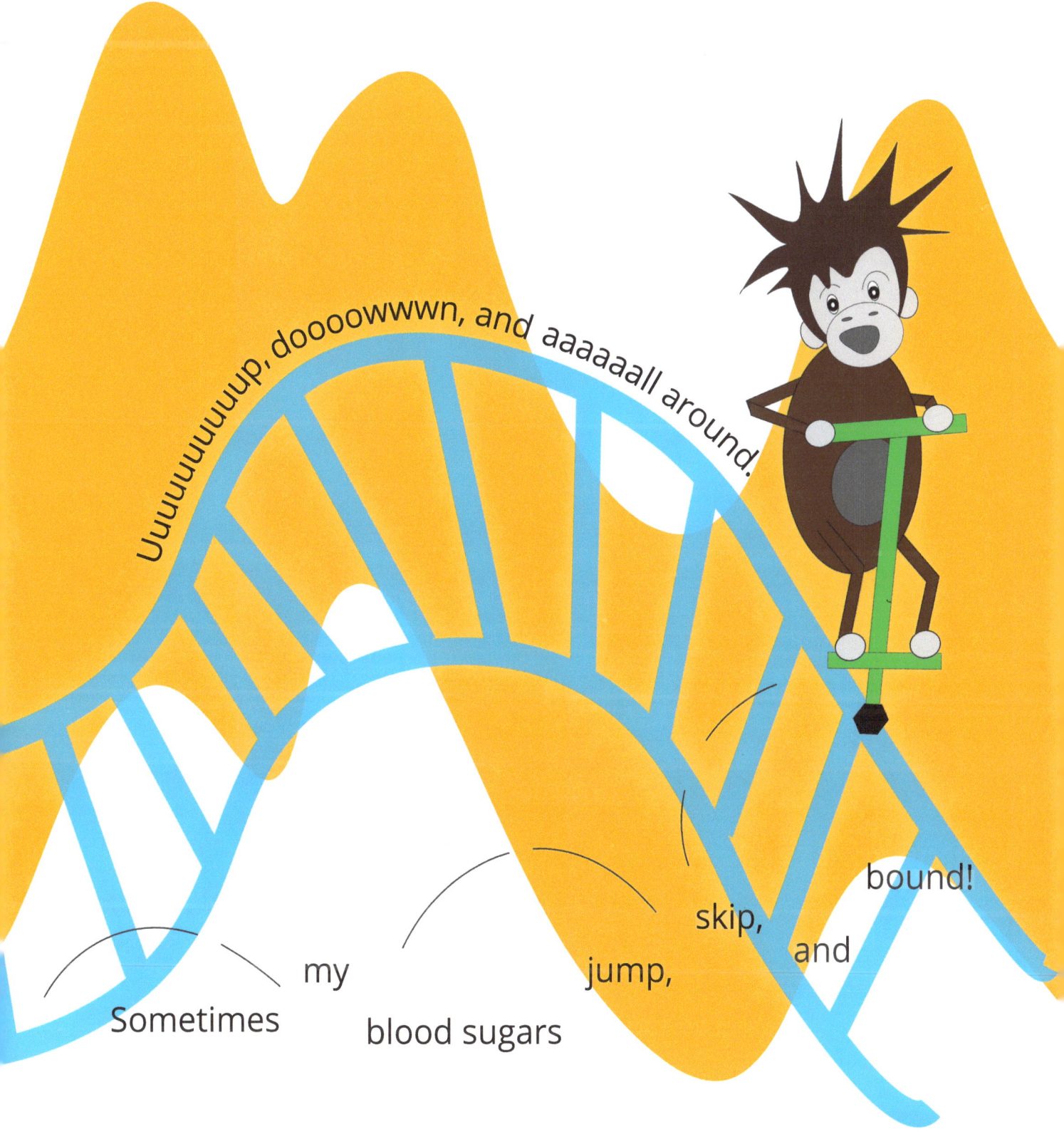

bound!

skip,

and

jump,

Sometimes

my

blood sugars

Sooo...,
what else do I have right here in my pack?
Insulin, of course—to keep me on track.

There're two types of insulin—one fast, one slow.
I take them both daily to stay on the go.

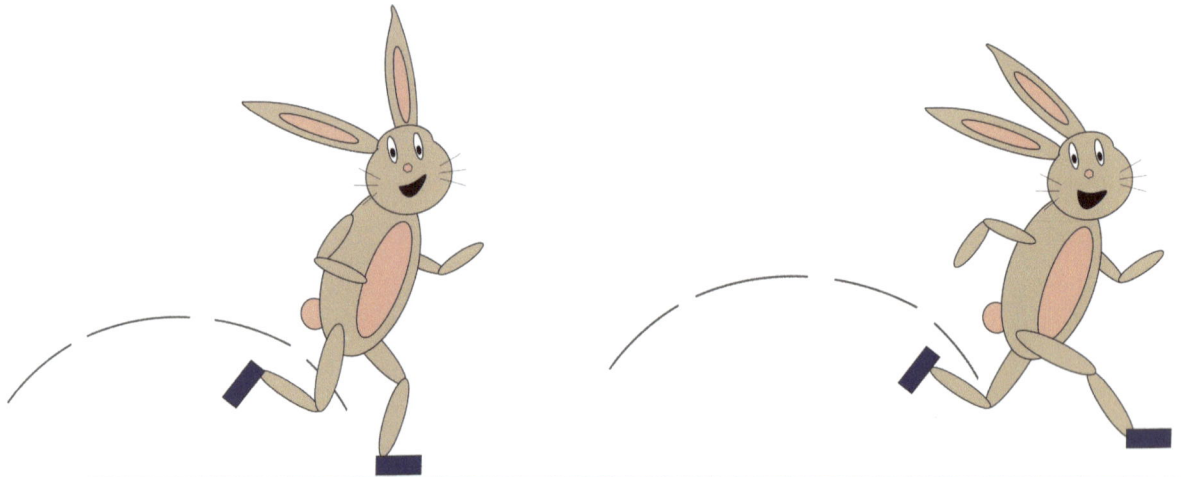

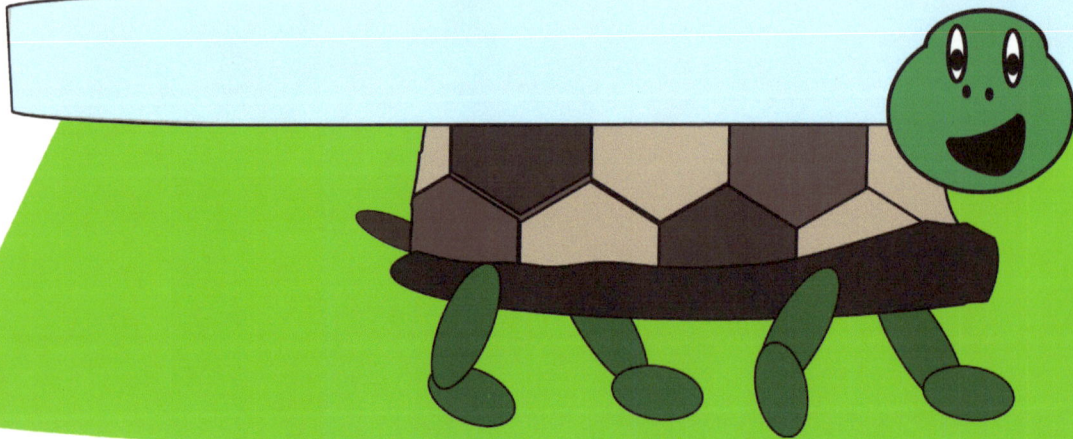

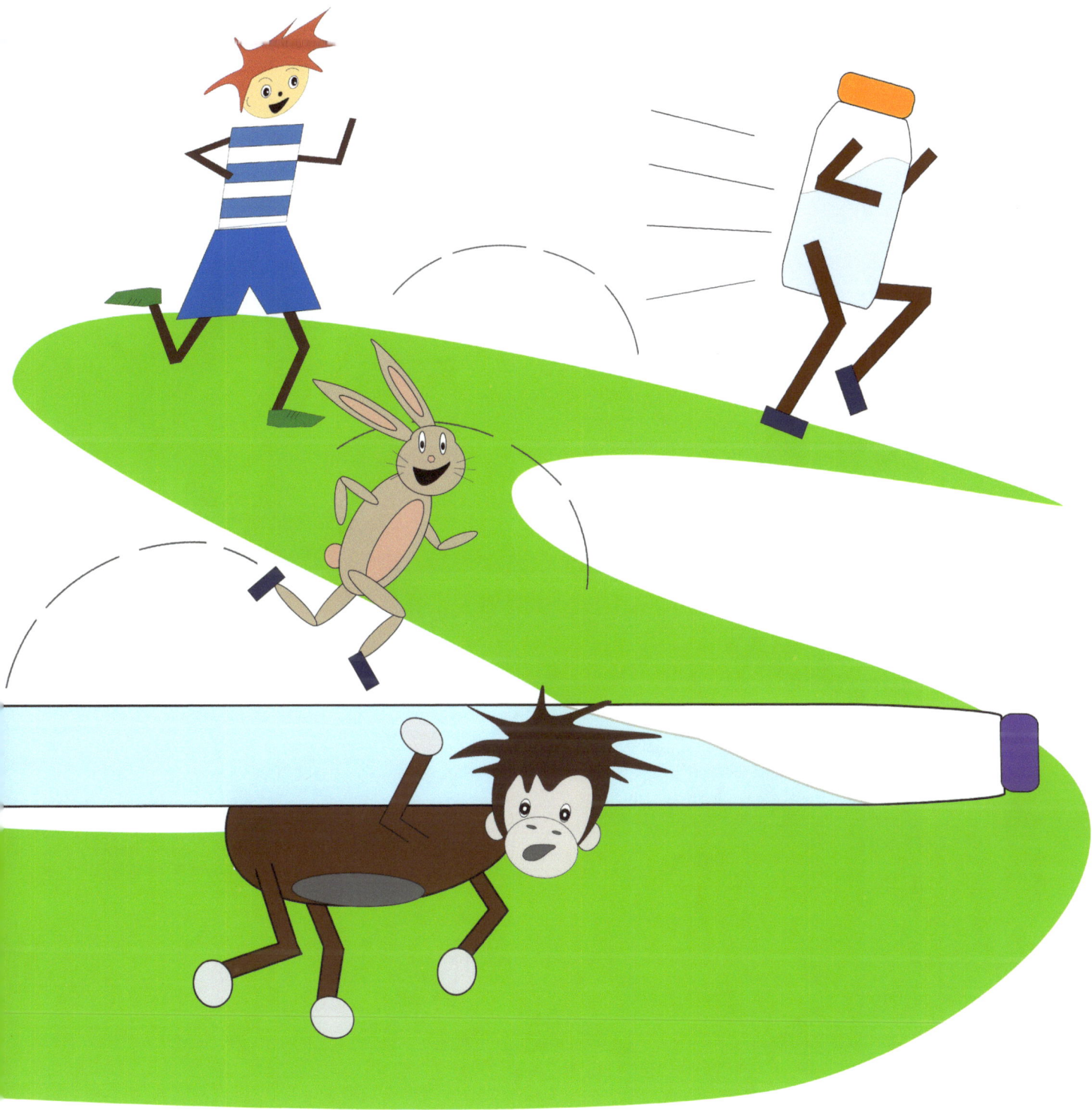

Together they mimic my old pancreas
to keep my blood sugar from running amiss.

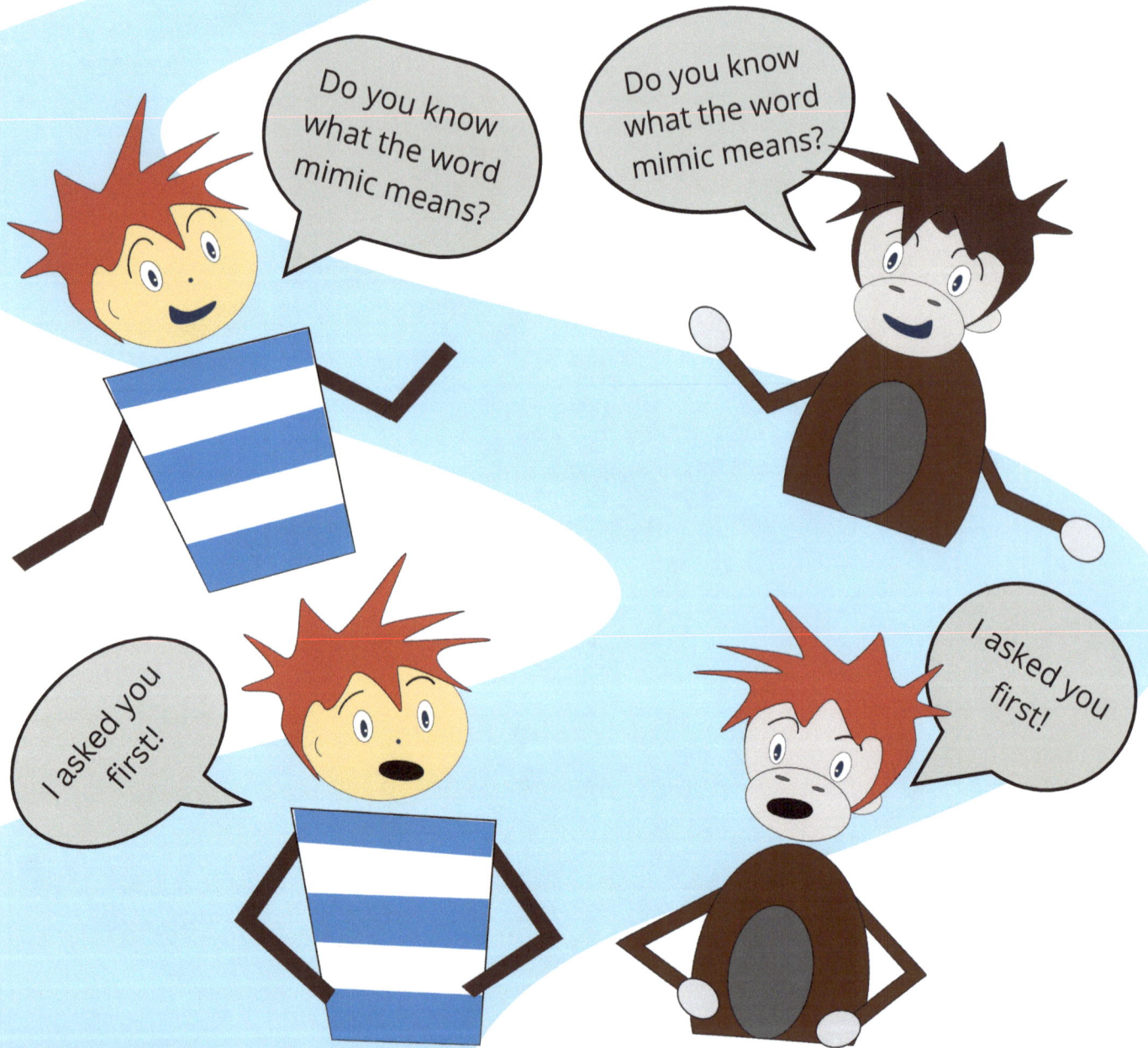

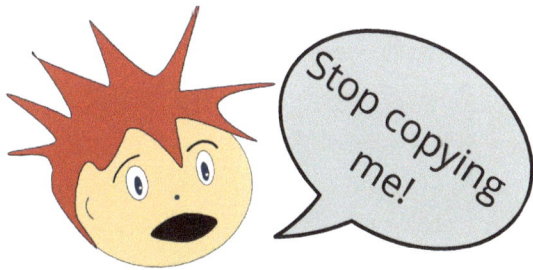

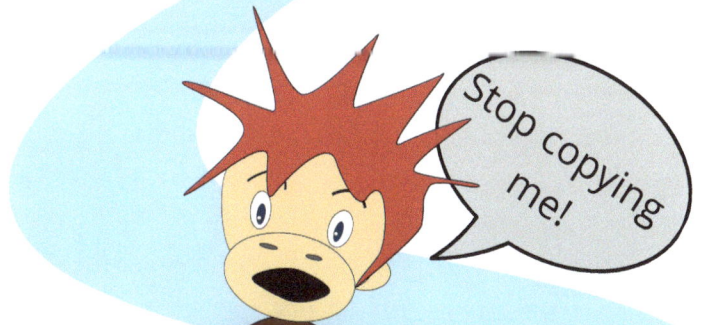

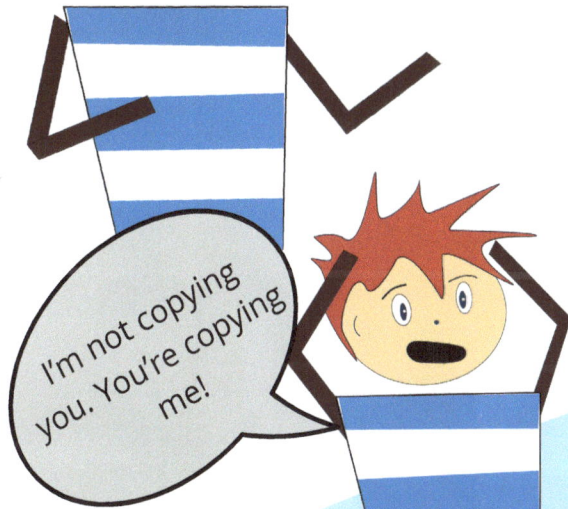

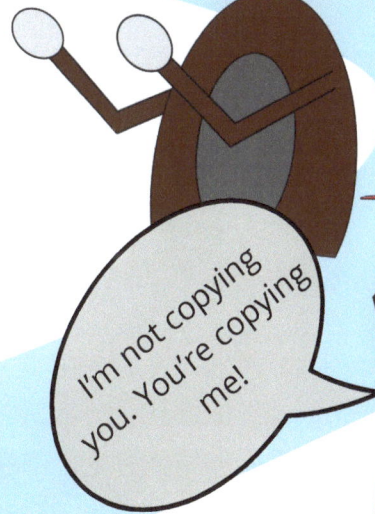

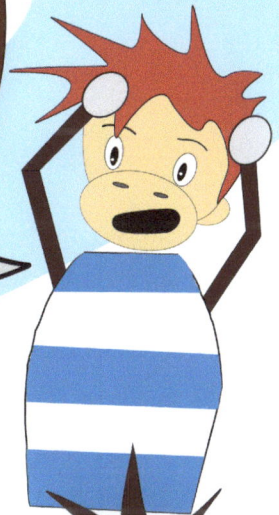

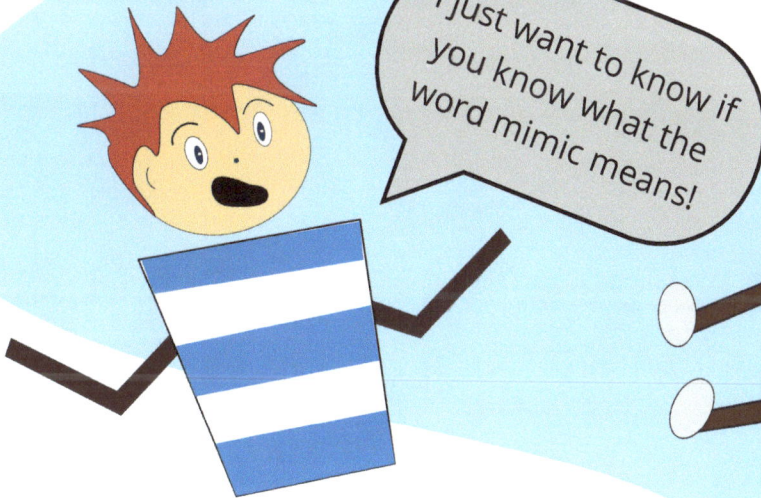

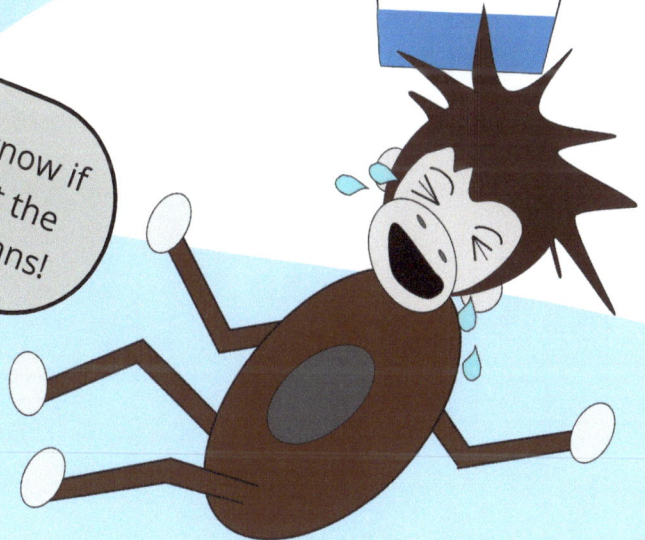

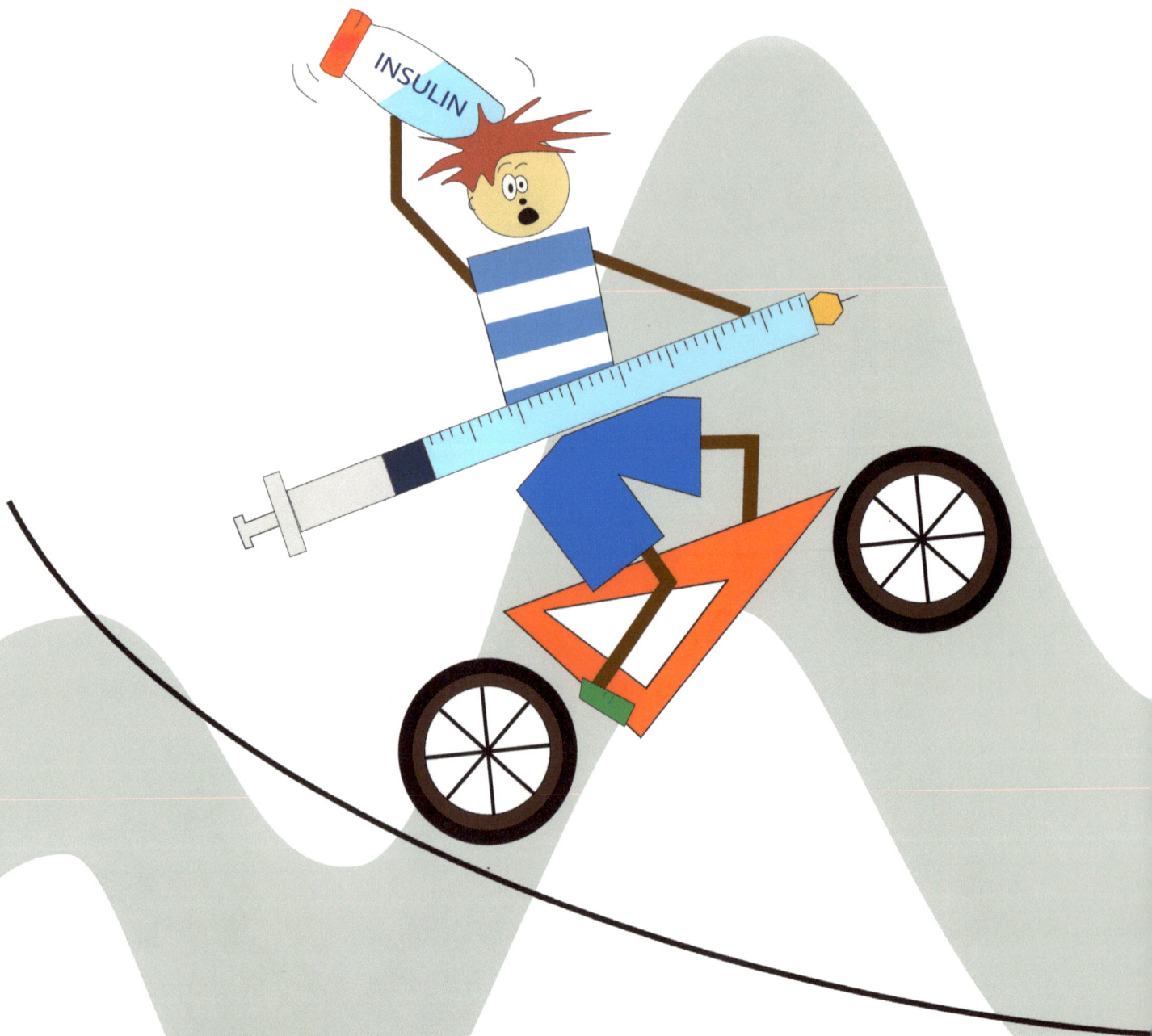

Slow-acting insulin I take once a day.
It steadies my sugars. At least, so they say.

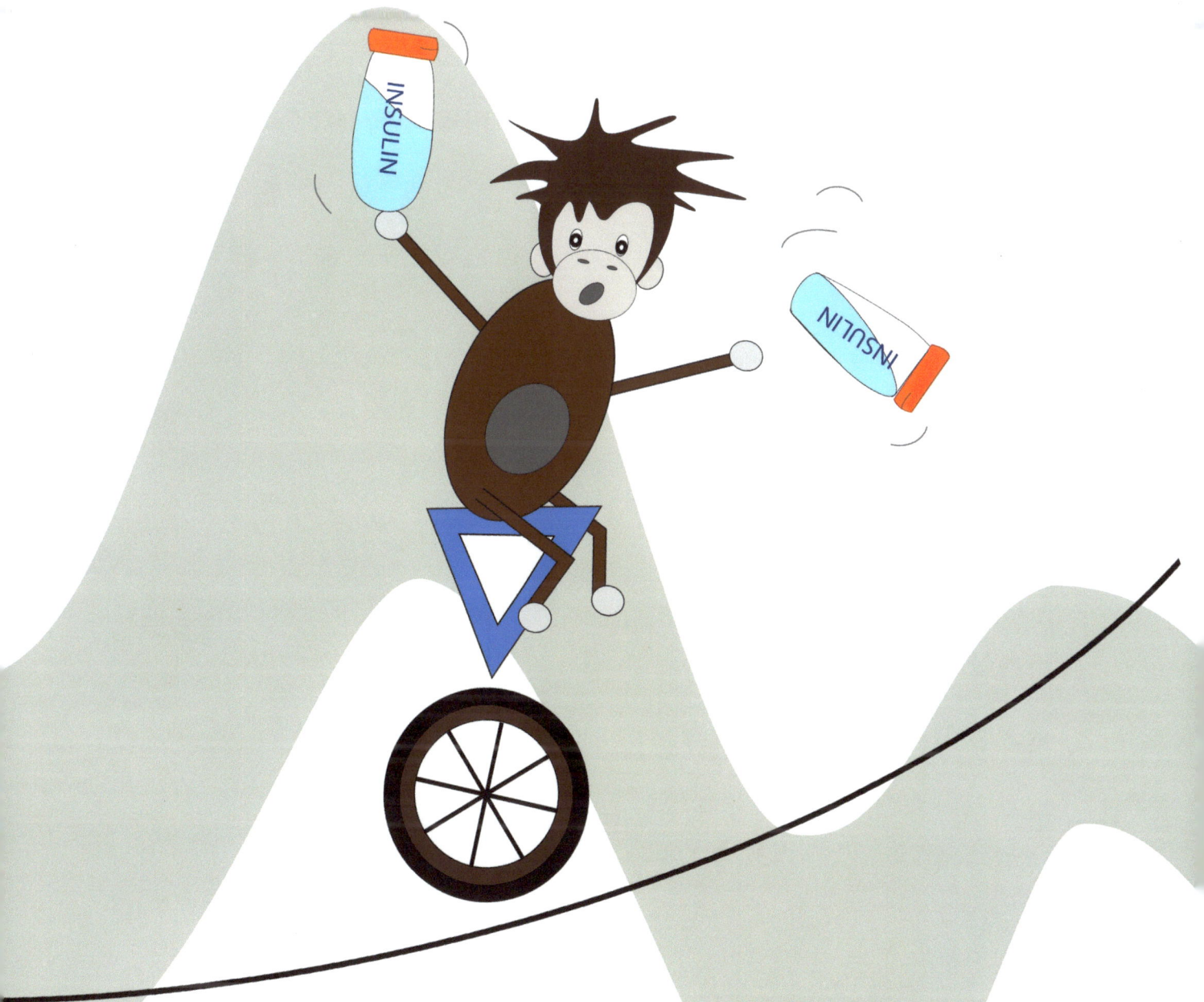

This insulin thing is a balancing act.
No doubt about it—and that is a fact!

Fast-acting insulin I take with my meals.
It stops my blood sugar from racing up hills.

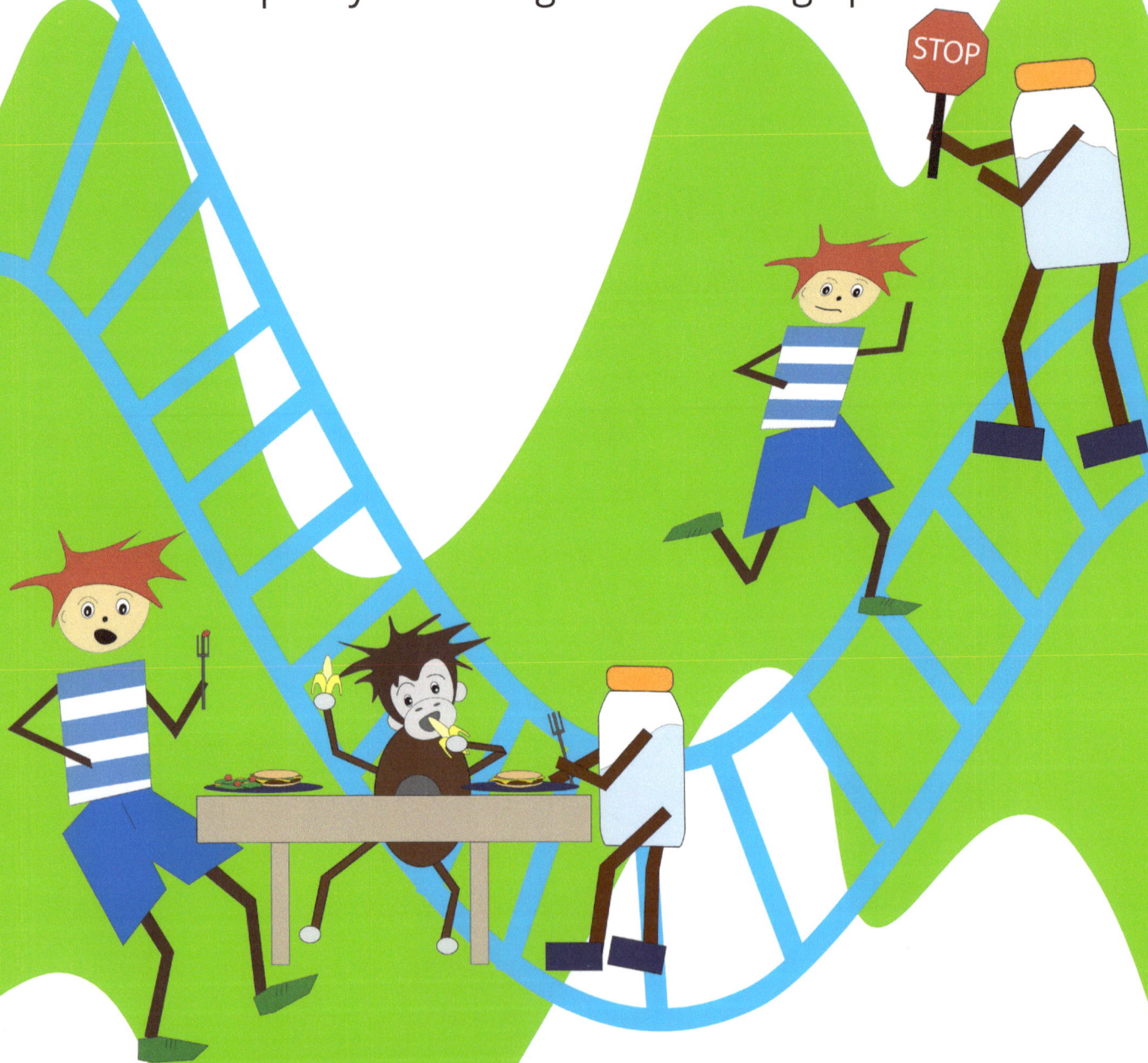

Sometimes I add just a little bit more,
if my sugar's too high and starting to soar.

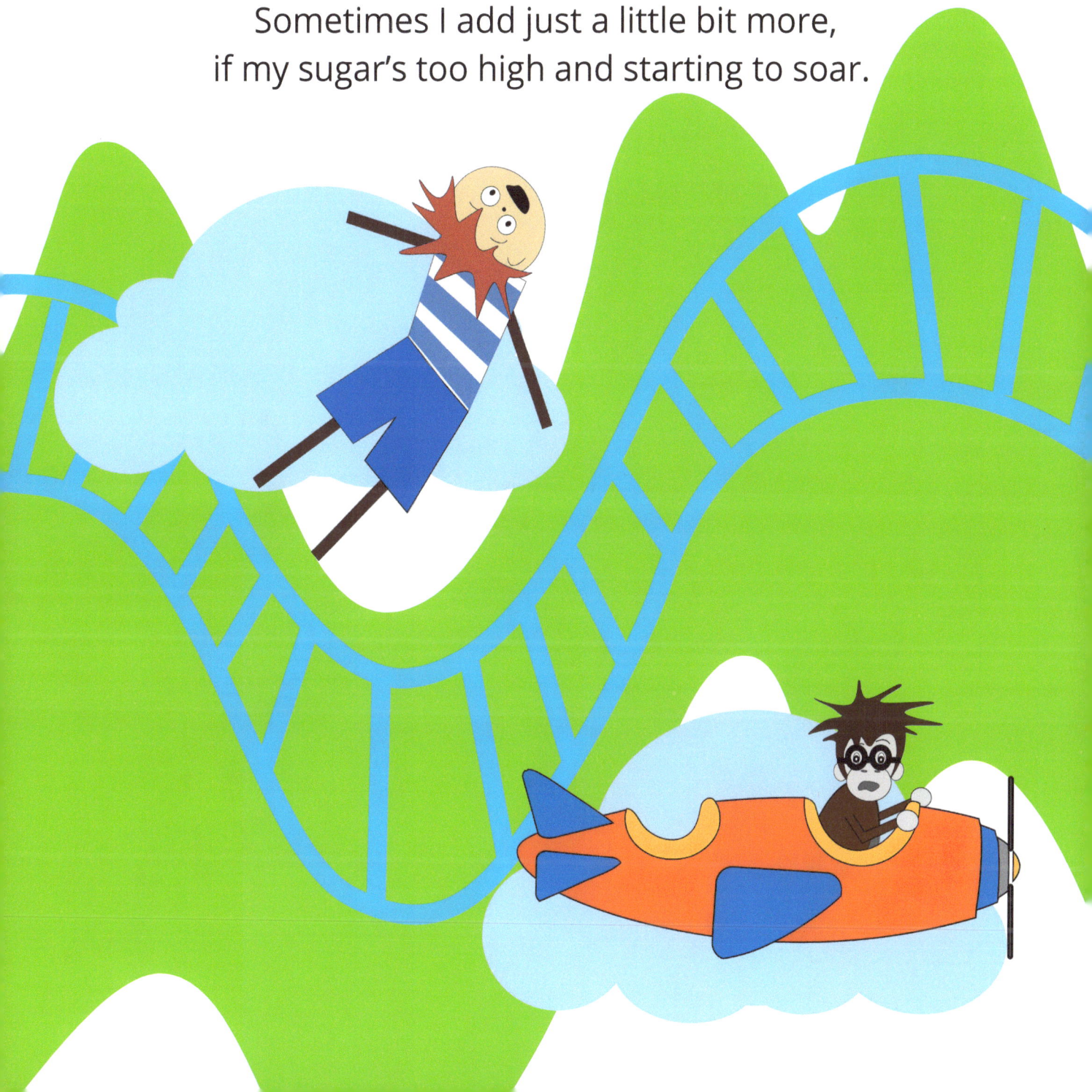

Blood sugar too high is nobody's treat.
Hyperglycemia's the worst kind of sweet.

What does it feel like? It's important to know!
It feels pretty gross from my head to my toe.

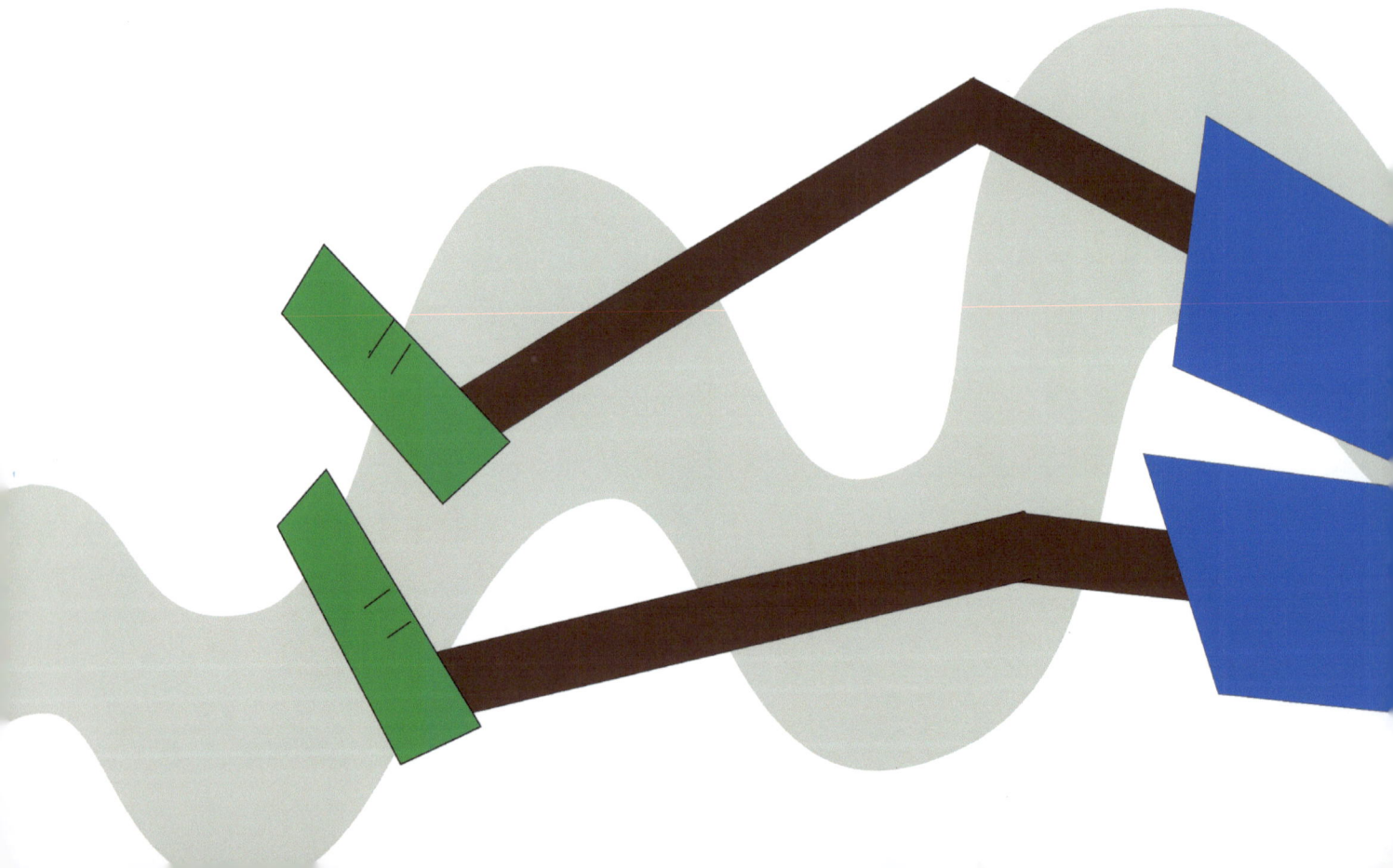

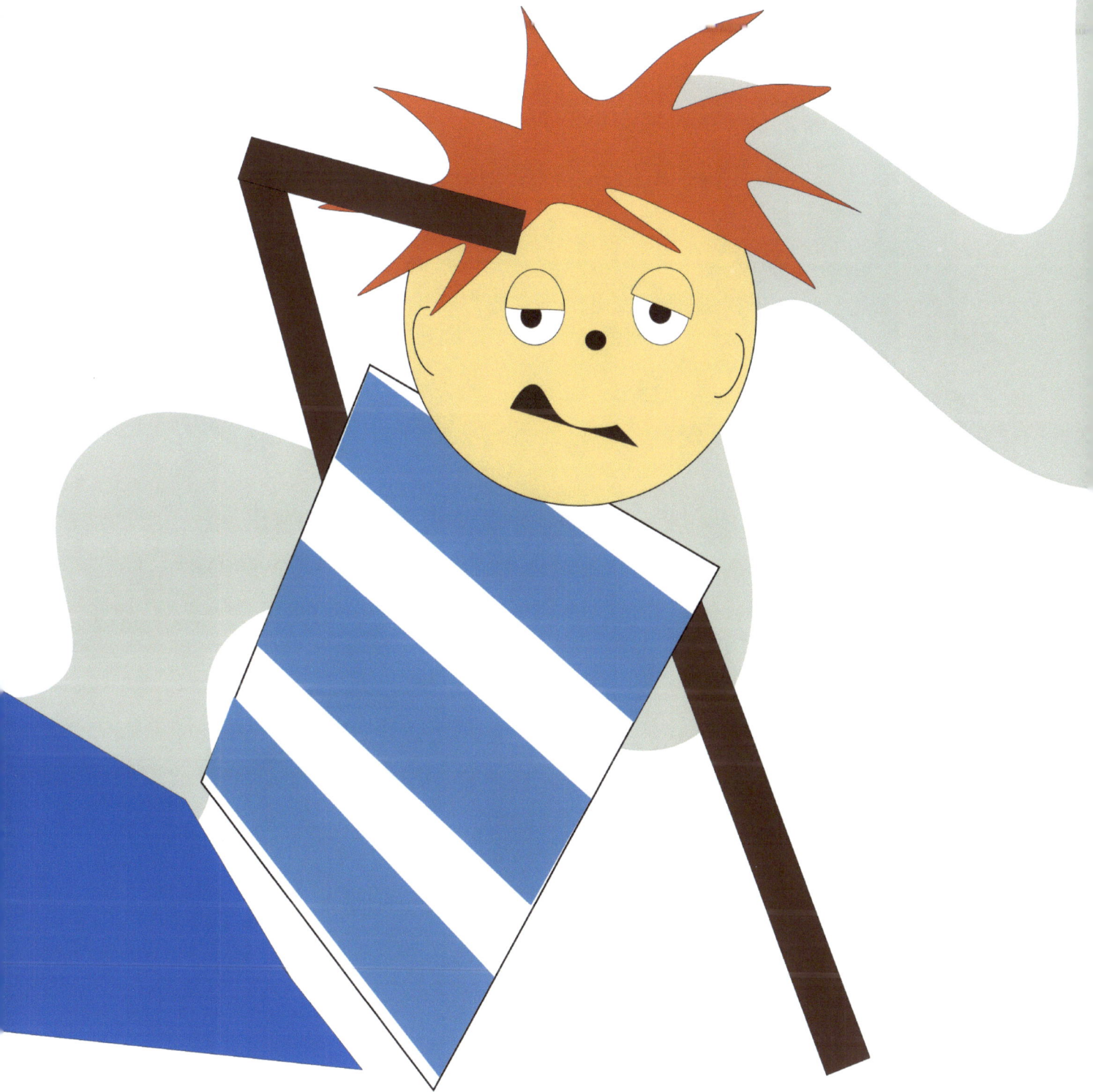

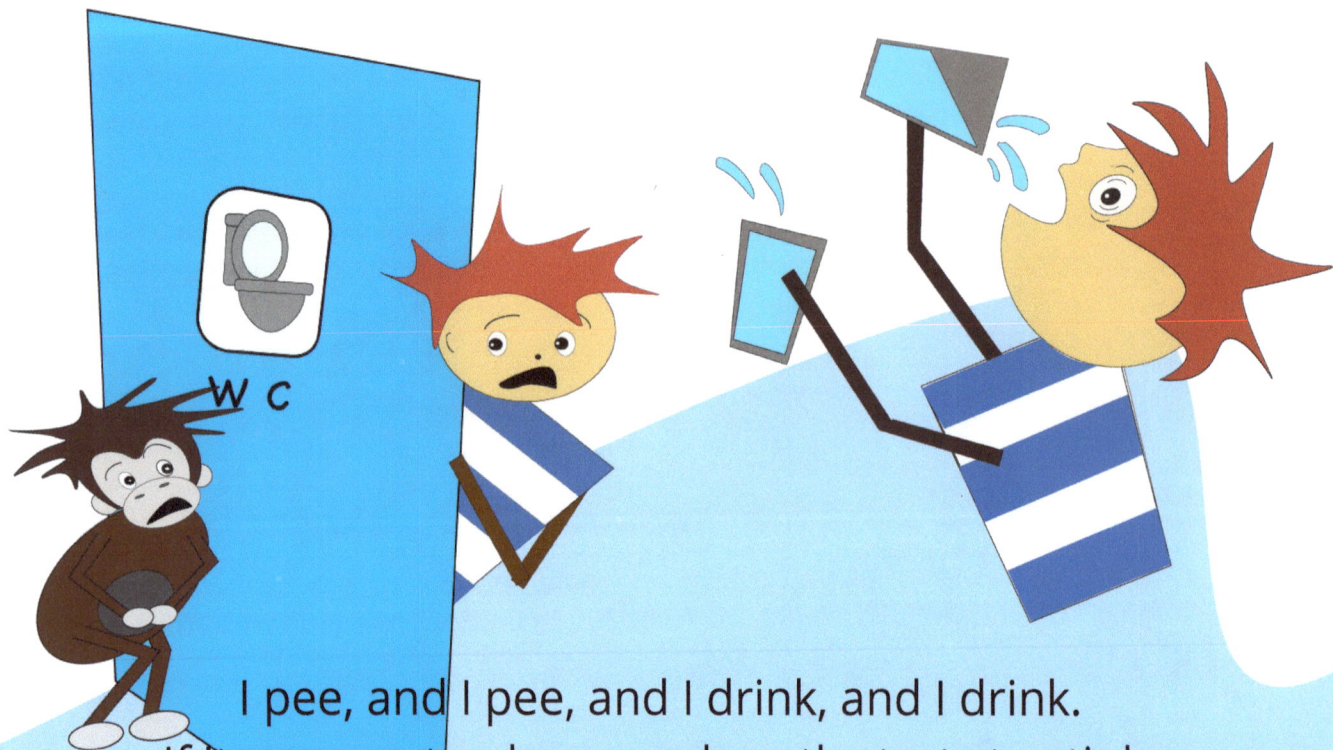

I pee, and I pee, and I drink, and I drink.
If it goes on too long, my breath starts to stink.

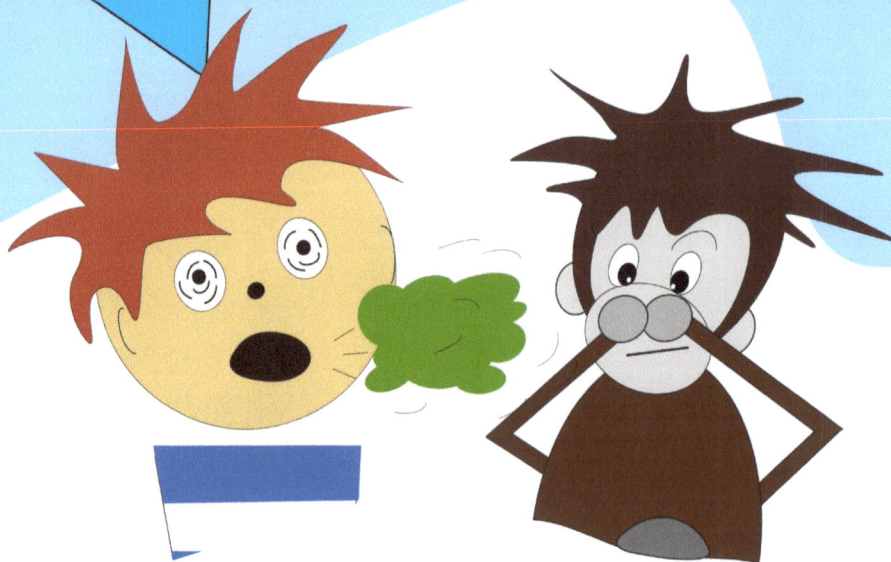

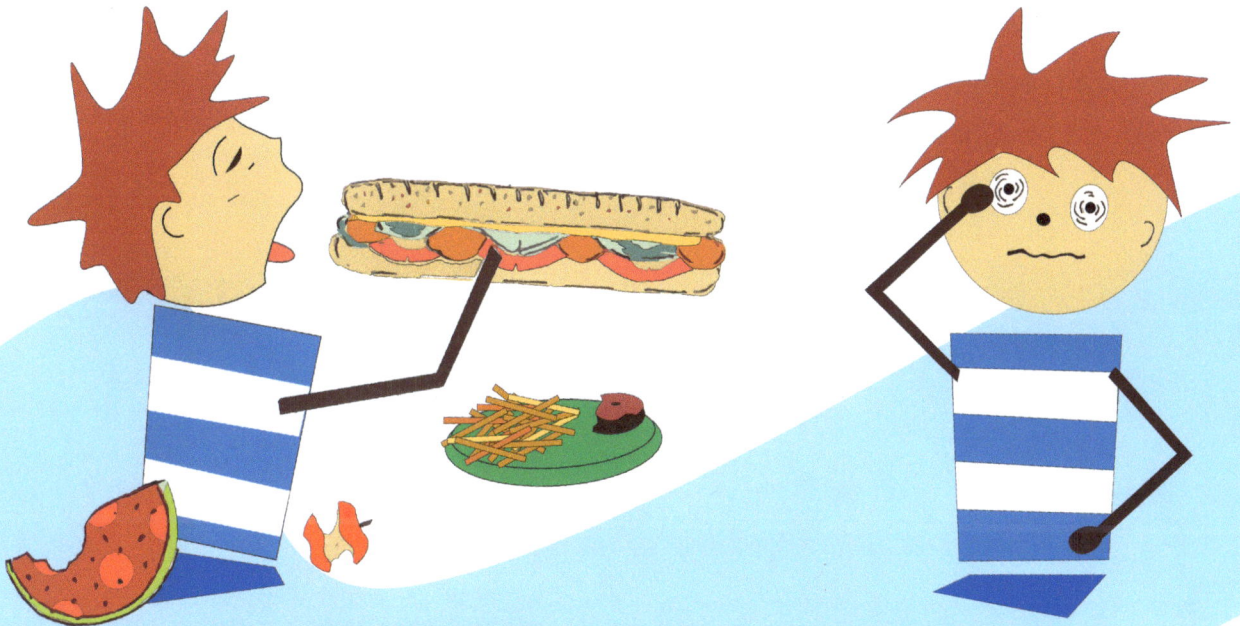

I get awf'lly hungry, and my eyes both blur.
My stomach starts hurting, and my brain won't whirr.

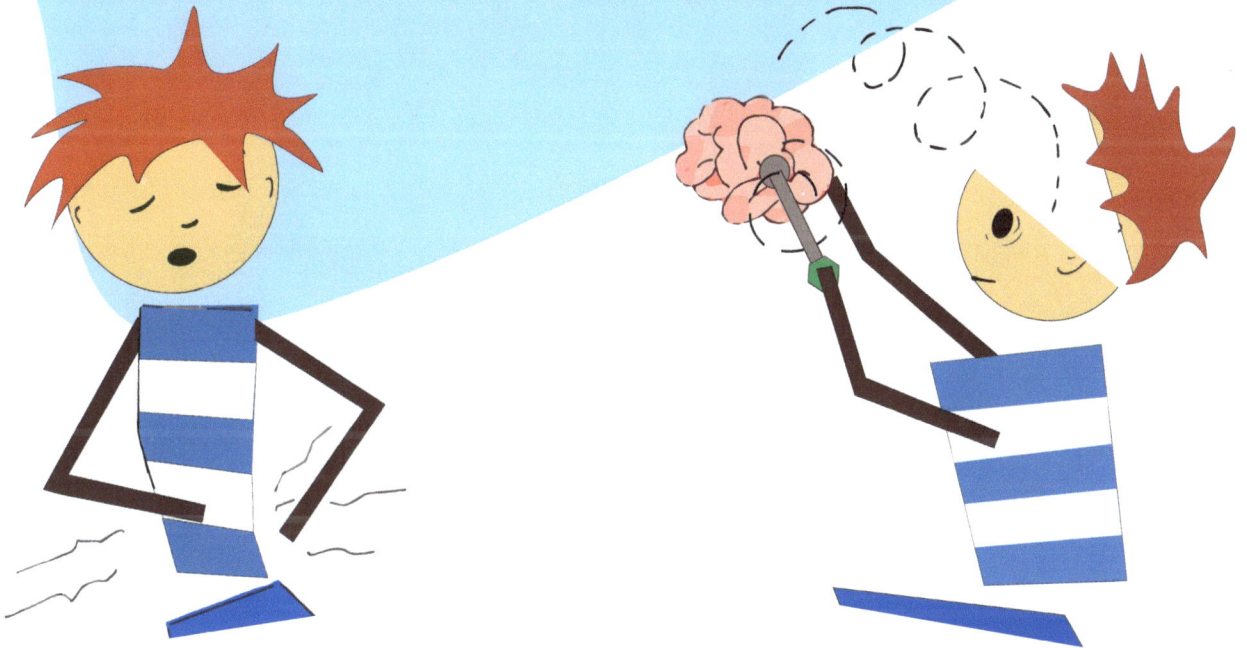

So, insulin's very important, you see,
to bring me back down to the me that is me.

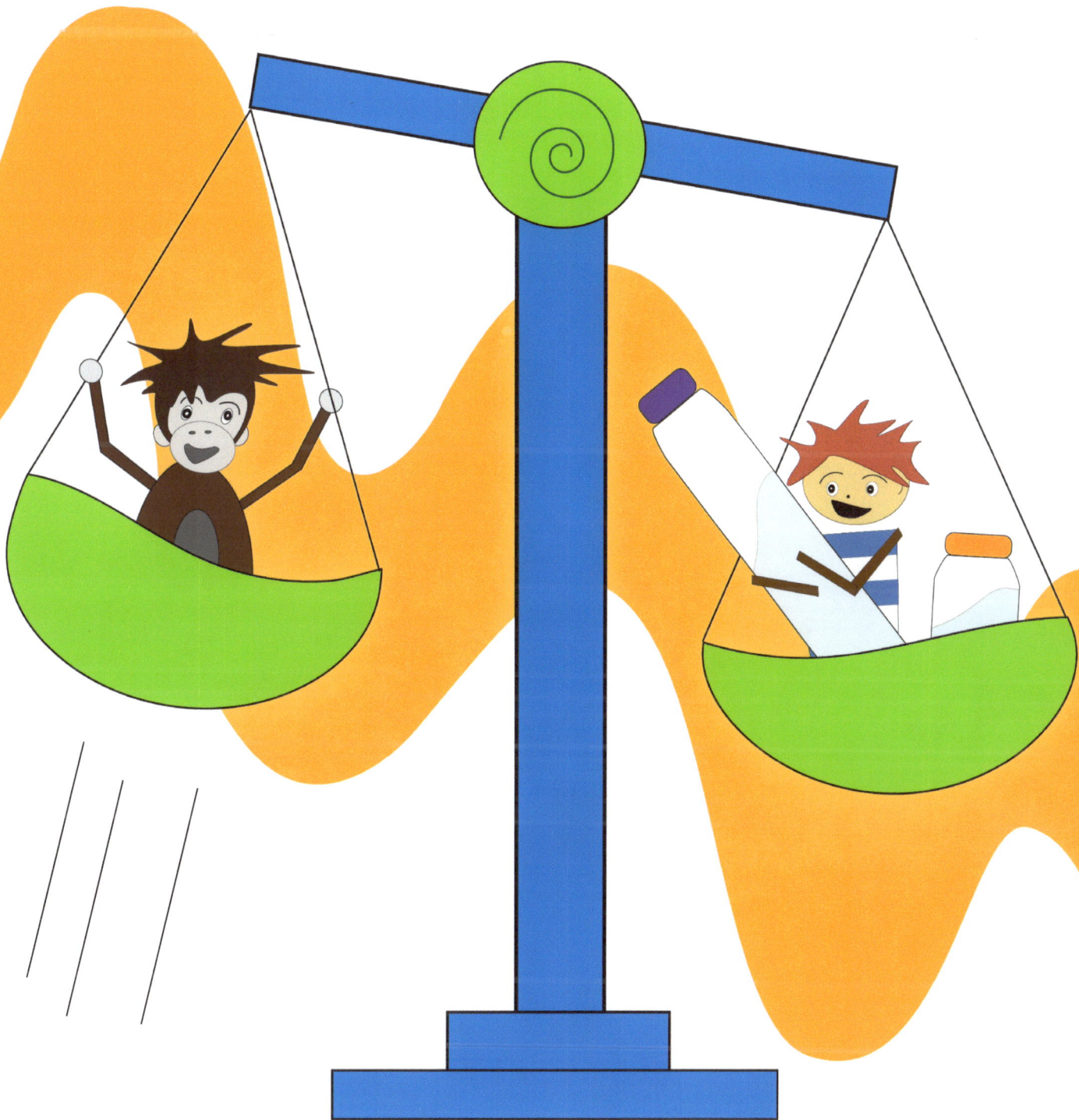

Blood sugars go high. Blood sugars go low. And I've got the skills to fix like a pro.

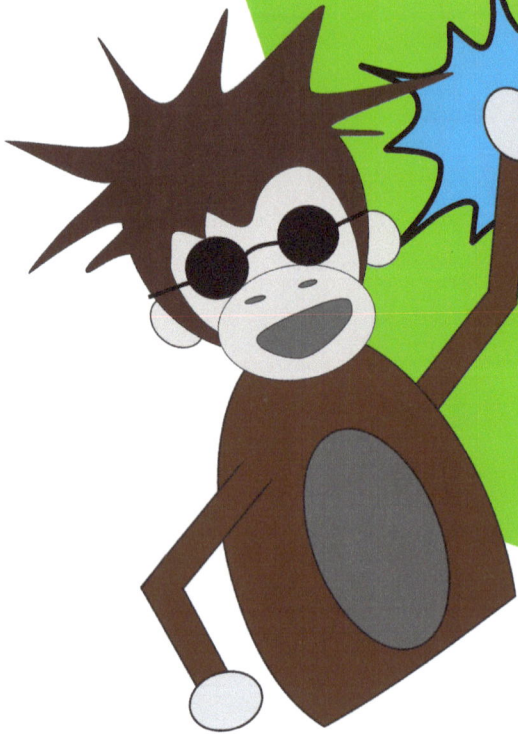

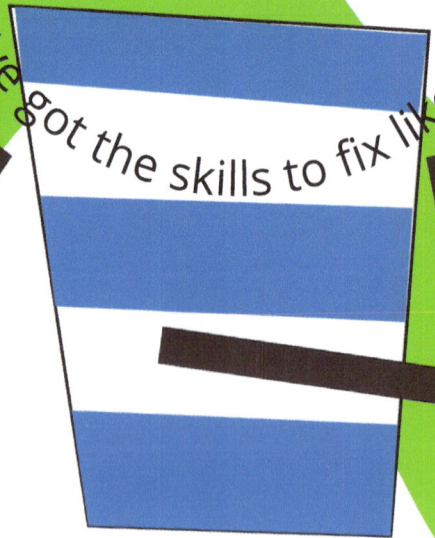

So, whether I'm up, or whether I'm down, steady and even, or all over town...

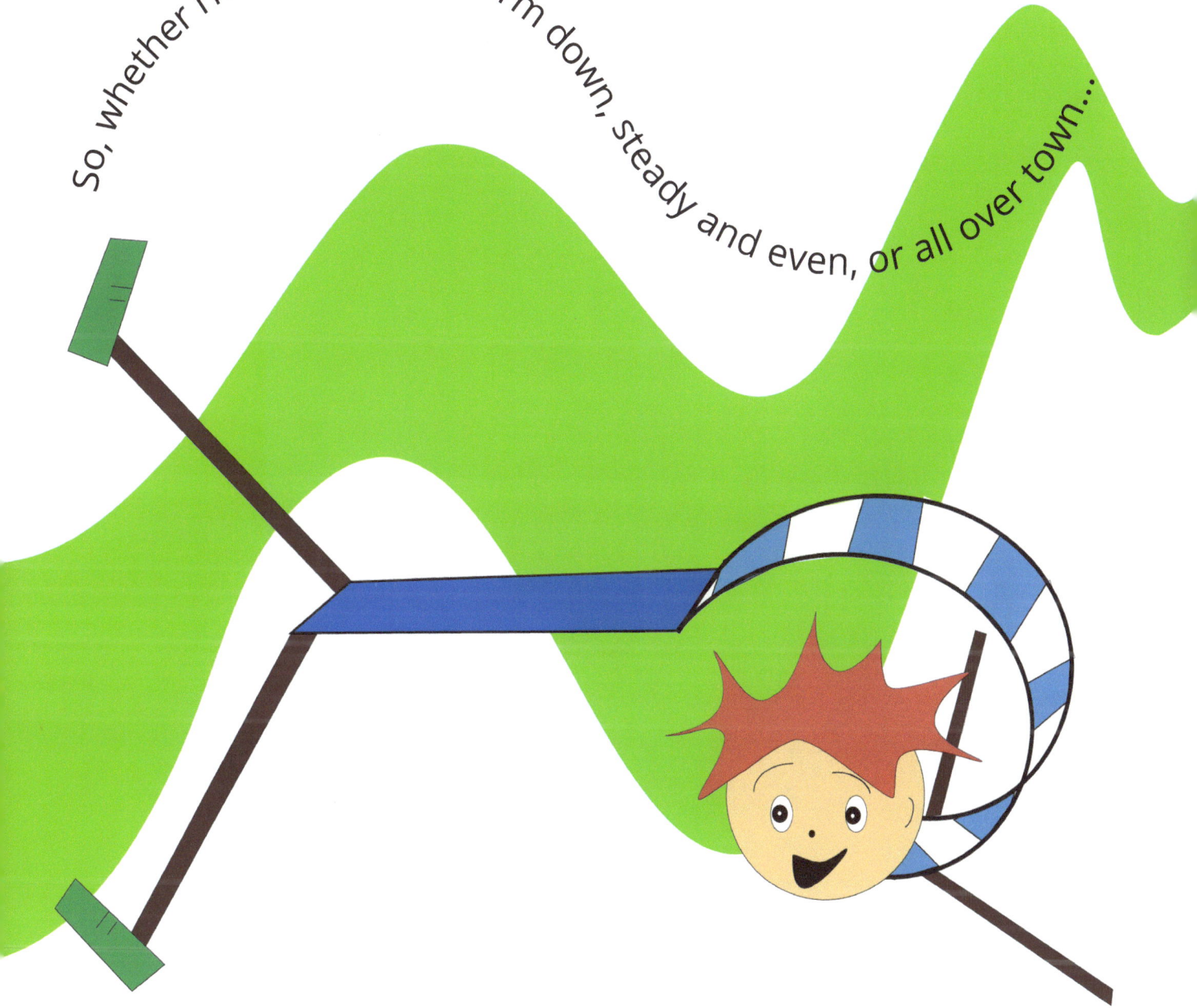

I can make the changes I need each day
to mend on the go, no matter which way.

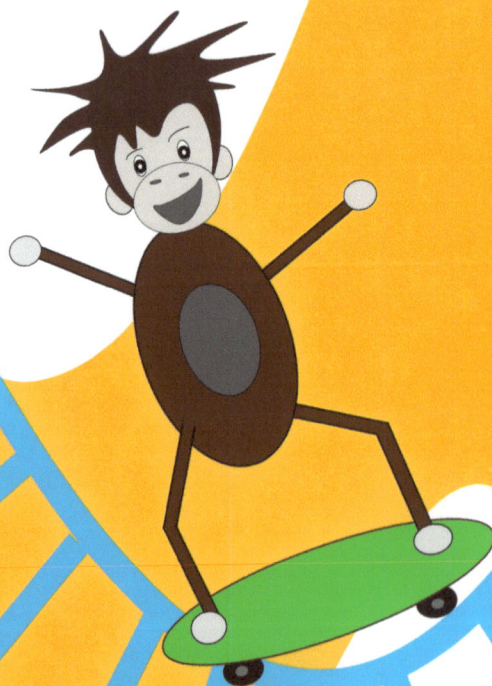

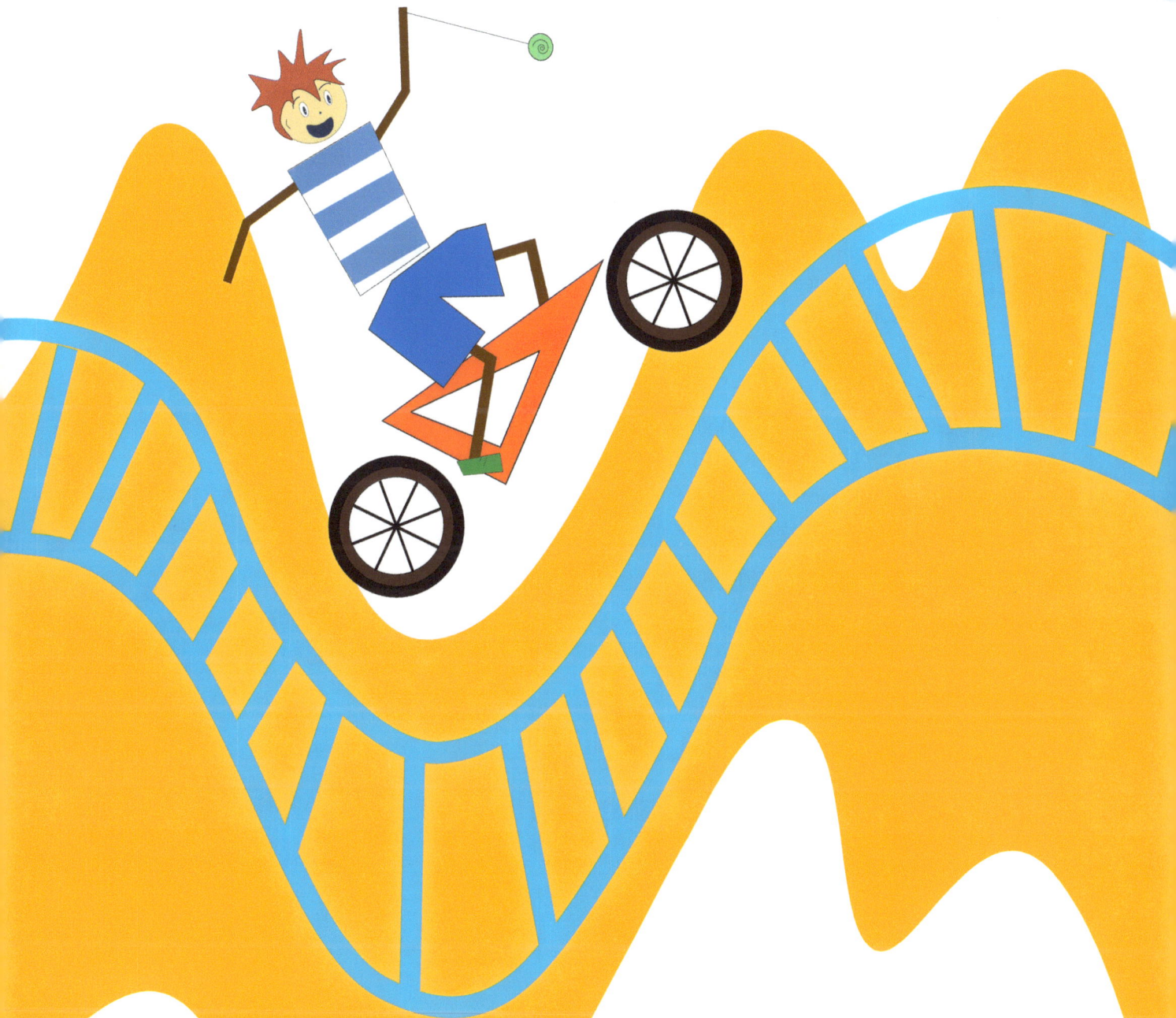

Hooray!

Tips for the Ride:

Treating Hypoglycemia:

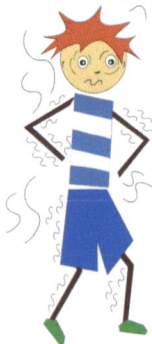

- If your blood sugar goes too low, you need a quick, simple carb snack.
- Simple carbs are things like fruit snacks, orange juice, hard candy, or glucose tablets.
- Signs of low blood sugar include feeling shaky, weak, dizzy, light-headed, sweaty, hungry, irritable, and/or nervous/anxious.
- Common causes of low blood sugar include taking too much insulin, eating too few carbs per insulin dose, waiting too long to eat after dosing insulin, or getting more physical activity than usual.

Treating Hyperglycemia:

- If your blood sugar goes too high, you need insulin.
- Your doctor will give you instructions on how to calculate your insulin dose.
- Signs of high blood sugar include drinking a lot, peeing a lot, blurry vision, and feeling hungry, tired, grumpy, and/or sick to your stomach.
- Common causes of high blood sugar include taking too little insulin, eating too many carbs per insulin dose, being sick, or getting less physical activity than usual.

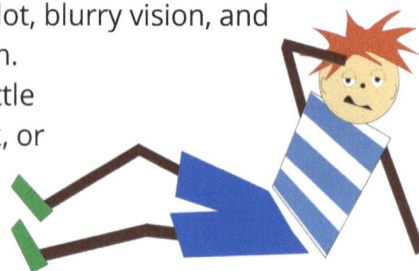

Mealtime Insulin Math:

Total units of Insulin $=$ units of insulin for your carbs $+$ units of insulin for your high blood sugar correction (if needed)

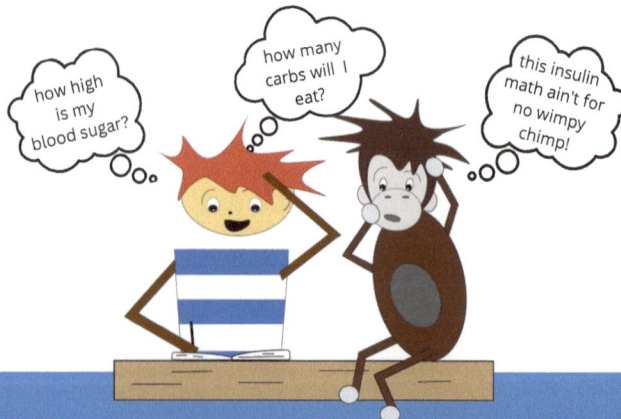

how high is my blood sugar?

how many carbs will I eat?

this insulin math ain't for no wimpy chimp!

Basal insulin:

Also called slow or long-acting insulin. This insulin is usually taken once a day. It works all day long to keep your blood sugars steady.

Bolus insulin:

Also called fast or short-acting insulin. This insulin is taken before meals to help keep your blood sugars from rising too much with food.

Carbohydrate:

Carbohydrates, or "carbs" for short, are foods that turn into sugar in your body.

Carb ratio:

This is for your mealtime insulin math. It tells you how much insulin you should take for a given amount of carbs. For example, if your carb ratio was 1:10, you would take 1 unit of short-acting insulin for every 10 grams of carbs you plan to eat.

Diabetic ketoacidosis (DKA):

DKA is a medical emergency that occurs when your body doesn't have enough insulin and your blood sugars get too high. Signs of DKA include increased thirst, frequent peeing, stomach pain, nausea, vomiting, fast breathing, confusion, fatigue, and fruity-smelling breath.

High glucose correction (HGC):

This number tells you how many points your blood sugar is expected to drop with one unit of fast-acting insulin. It is part of your mealtime insulin math. If your blood sugar is too high at mealtime, you can use your HGC to help bring it back down to where it belongs.

Rule of 15s:

If your blood sugar level goes below your target range, eat 15 grams of carbs, wait 15 min, and then recheck your blood sugar. Repeat, as needed, until your blood sugar is back in range.

Special thanks to all of my beta readers. Your fingerprints are all over this book.

The art for this book is inspired by construction paper cutouts. Any kid could do it. A chimpanzee probably could too.

Also written by Amelia:

Was it Something I Ate? The Type 1 Diabetes Myth Buster for Kids

Note to the reader:

The content in this book is for educational and informational purposes only and is based on widely published research available to the author. The content should not be considered a substitute for professional medical advice. Please consult regularly with your medical provider for the most up-to-date and appropriate treatment guidelines for you.

www.ingramcontent.com/pod-product-compliance
Lightning Source LLC
Chambersburg PA
CBHW041546260326
41914CB00016B/1567